Current Topics in Neglected Tropical Diseases

Edited by Alfonso J. Rodriguez-Morales

Published in London, United Kingdom

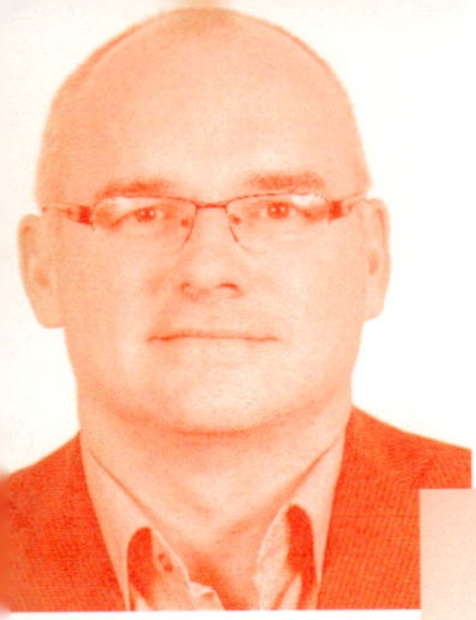
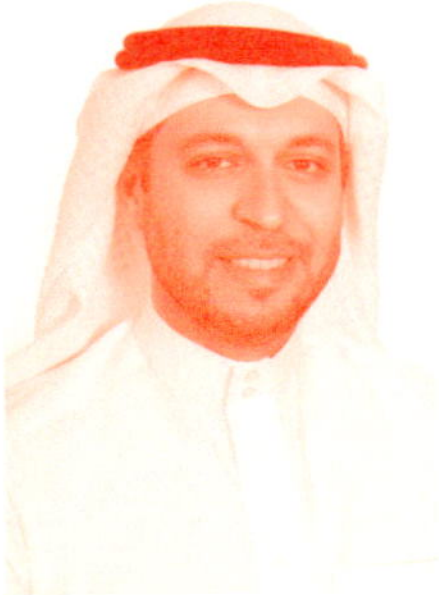
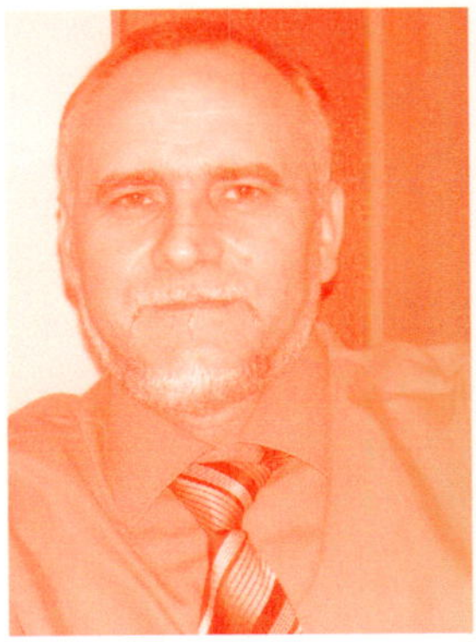
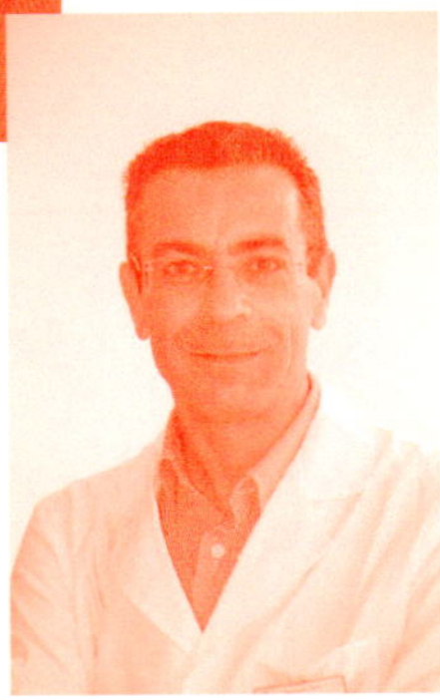
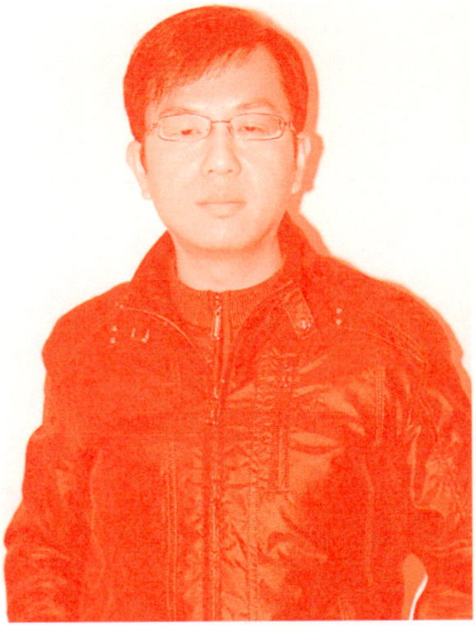
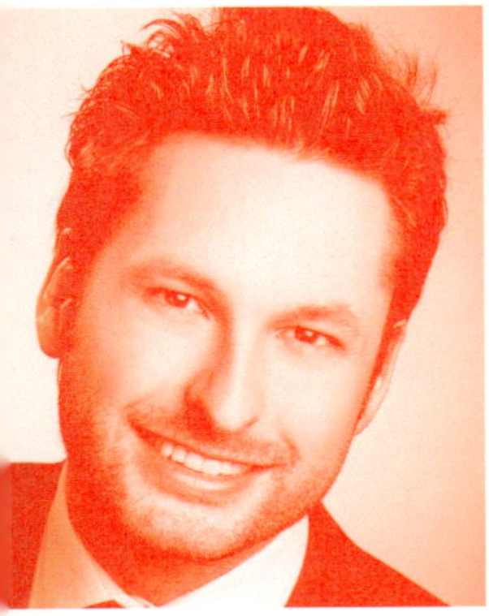
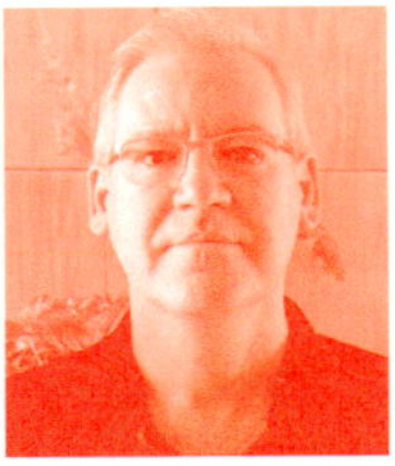

IntechOpen

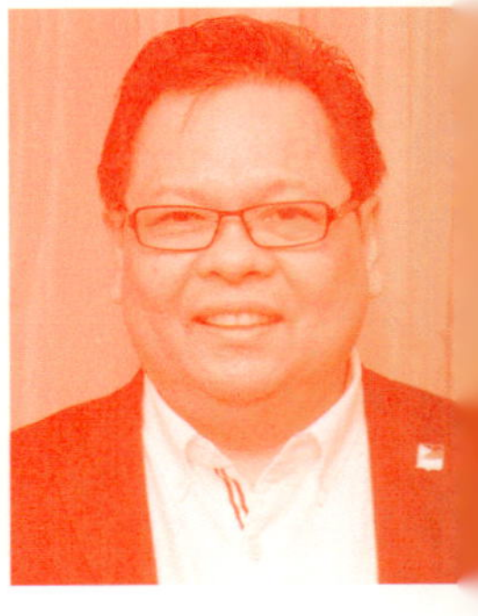
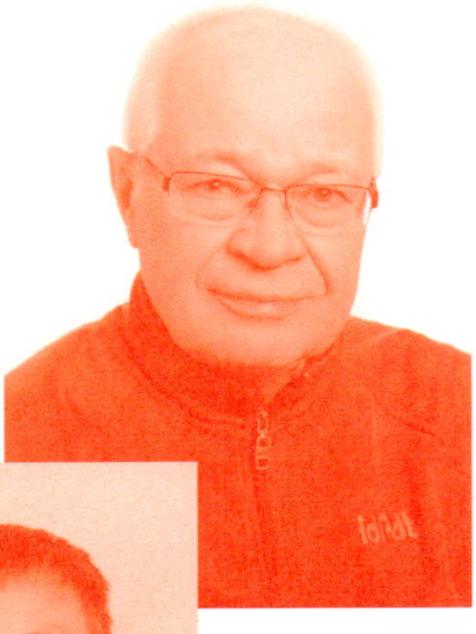
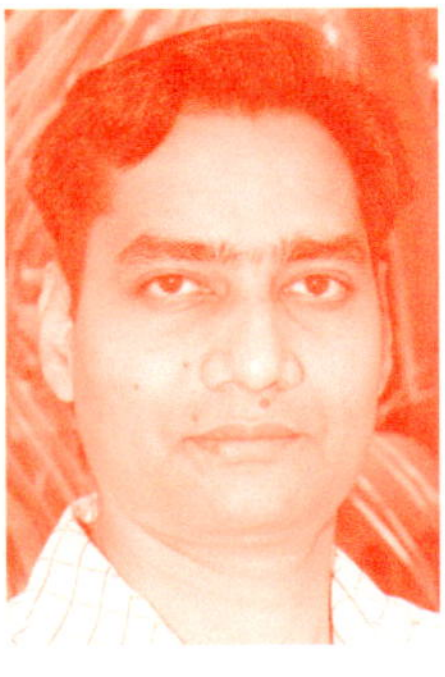
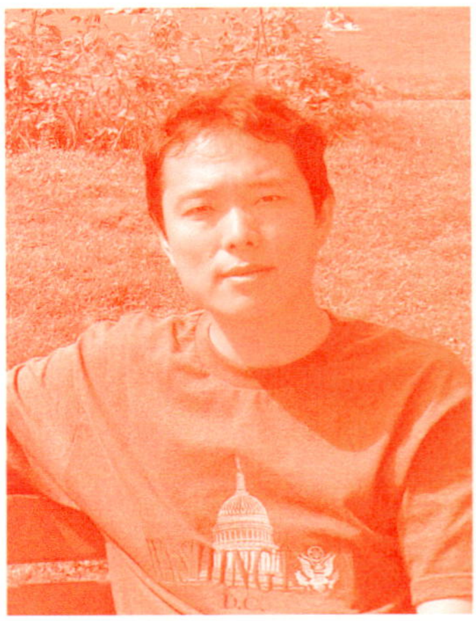
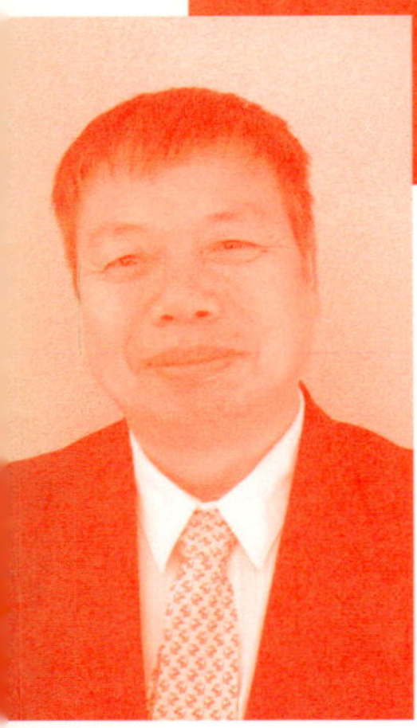
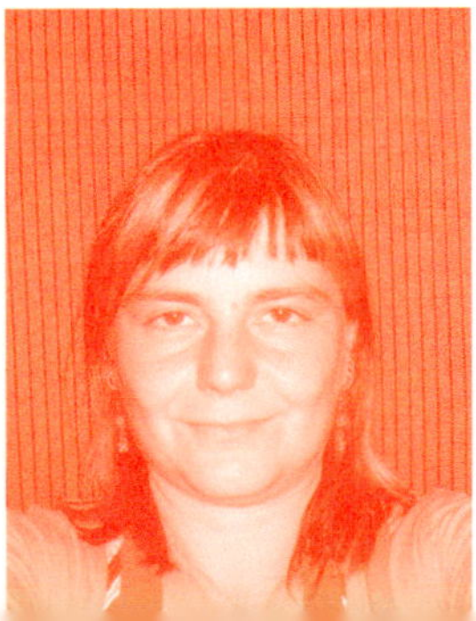

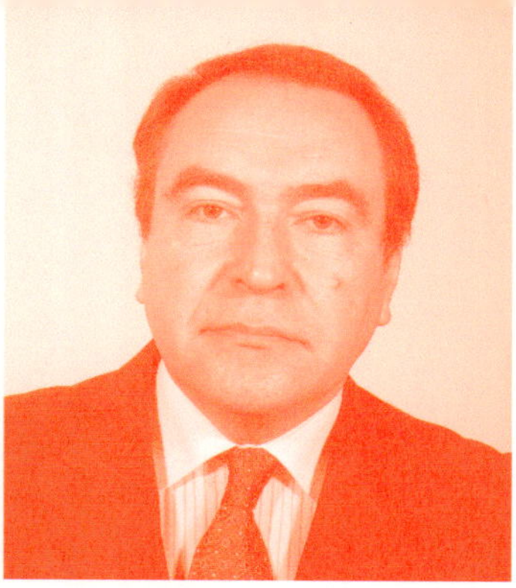
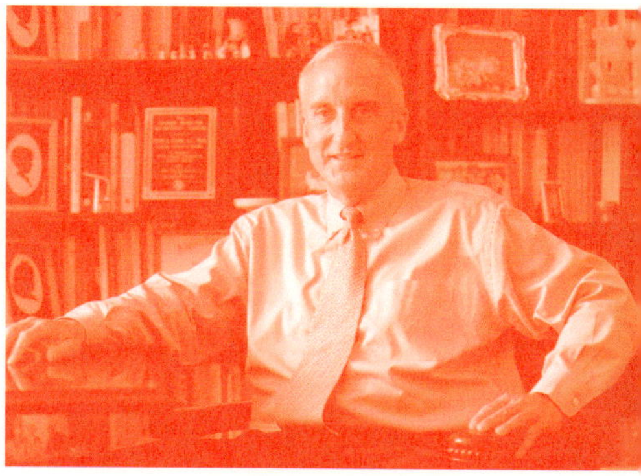
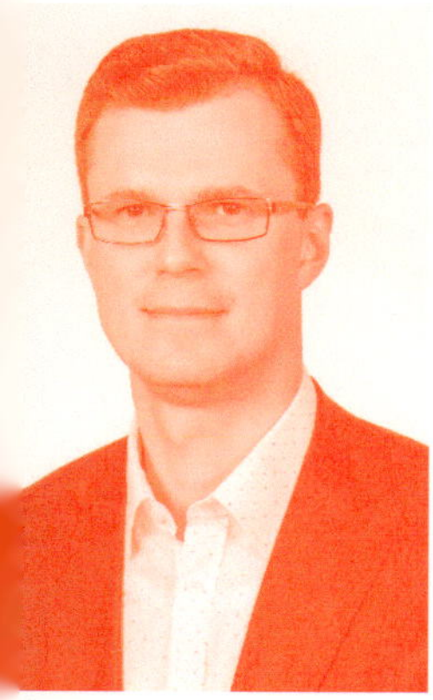
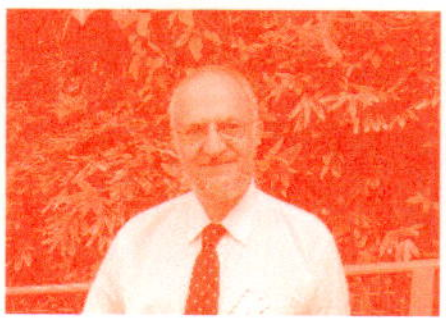
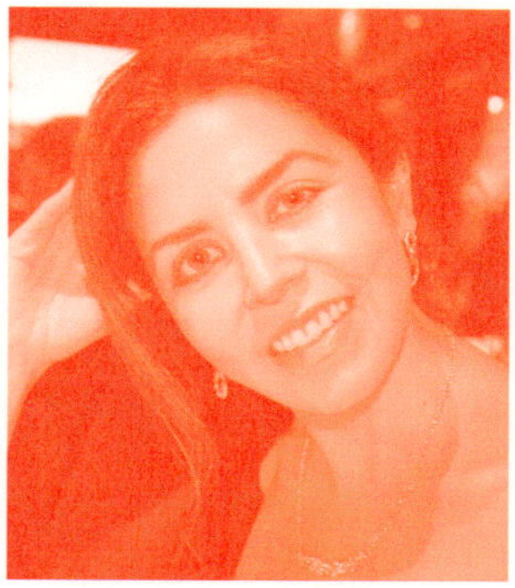

Supporting open minds since 2005

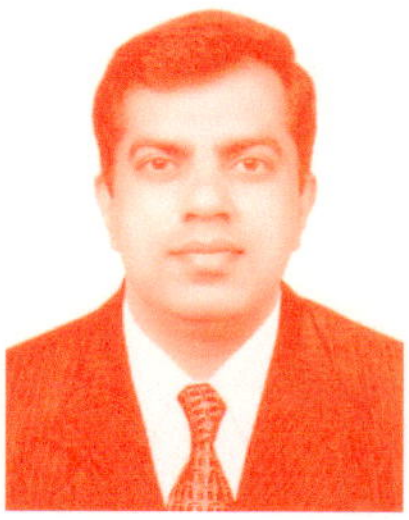
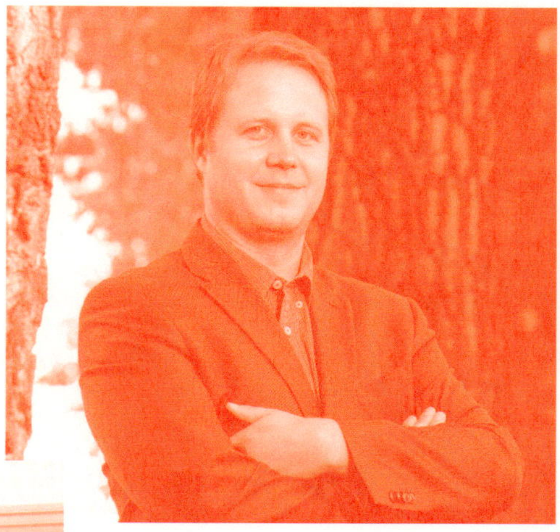
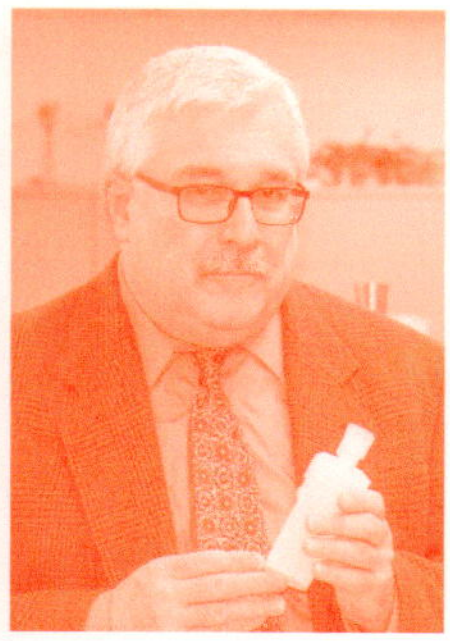
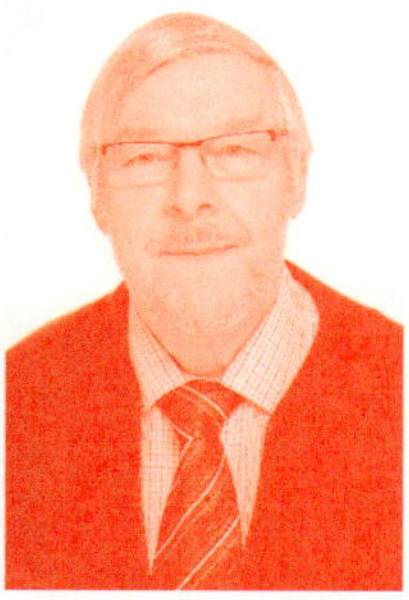
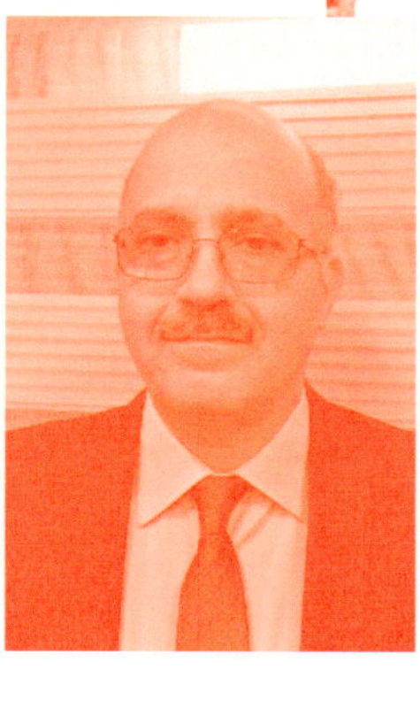
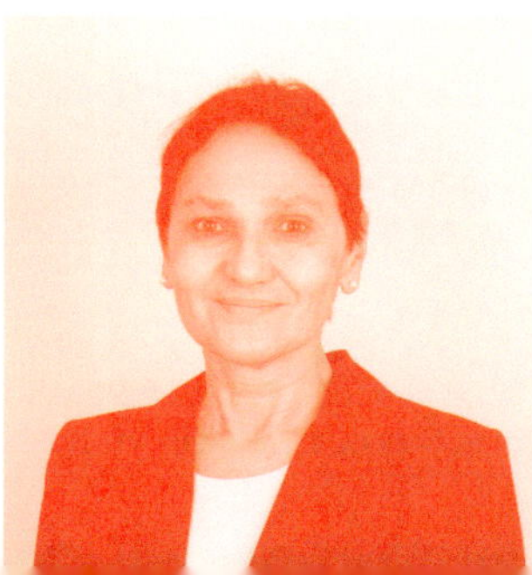
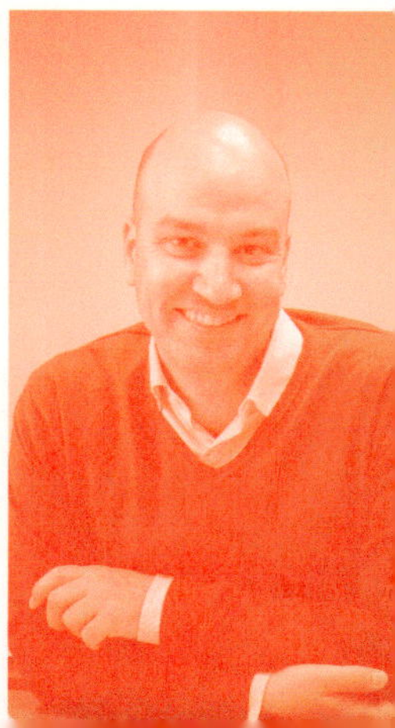

Current Topics in Neglected Tropical Diseases
http://dx.doi.org/10.5772/intechopen.73918
Edited by Alfonso J. Rodriguez-Morales

Part of IntechOpen Book Series: Infectious Diseases, Volume 3
Book Series Editor: Shailendra K. Saxena

Contributors
Imelda K. K Moise, Leo C. Zulu, Douglas O. Fuller, John C. Beier, Marta E. Álvarez-Argüelles, Susana Rojo Alba, Jose Antonio Boga Riveiro, Santiago Melón García, Mercedes Rodríguez Pérez, Tonay Inceboz, Joshua Britton Bilsborrow, Robert T. Schoen, José Kennedy Amaral, Debajanee Lenka, Amarendra Mohapatra, Chittaranjan Kar, Shailendra K. Saxena, Angel Ramos-Ligonio, Aracely López-Monteon, Eric Dumonteil, Tran Hau Khang, Ngo Minh Thao, Le Huu Doanh, Issiaka Soulama

First published in London, United Kingdom, 2019 by IntechOpen
IntechOpen is the global imprint of INTECHOPEN LIMITED, registered in England and Wales, registration number: 11086078, 7th floor, 10 Lower Thames Street, London, EC3R 6AF, United Kingdom
Printed in Croatia

British Library Cataloguing-in-Publication Data
A catalogue record for this book is available from the British Library

Additional hard and PDF copies can be obtained from orders@intechopen.com

Current Topics in Neglected Tropical Diseases
Edited by Alfonso J. Rodriguez-Morales
p. cm.
Print ISBN 978-1-78923-889-1
Online ISBN 978-1-78923-890-7
eBook (PDF) ISBN 978-1-78984-143-5

For EU product safety concerns:
IN TECH d.o.o., Prolaz Marije Krucifikse Kozulić 3, 51000 Rijeka, Croatia, info@intechopen.com or visit our website at intechopen.com.

IntechOpen Book Series
Infectious Diseases
Volume 3

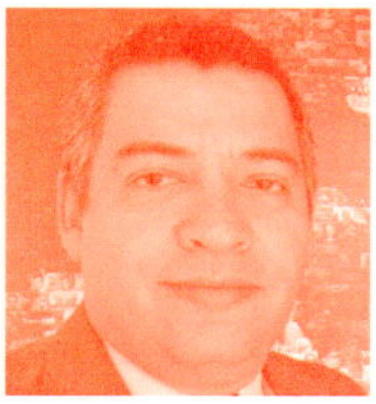

Dr. Alfonso J. Rodriguez-Morales received his Doctor of Medicine (MD) degree from Universidad Central de Venezuela, Caracas, and his Master of Sciences in Protozoology (MSc) from Universidad de Los Andes, Trujillo, Venezuela. He received his Diploma in Tropical Medicine & Hygiene (DTM&H) from Universidad Peruana Cayetano Heredia, Lima, Peru, and University of Alabama at Birmingham, Birmingham, Alabama, USA. He is a Fellow of the Royal Society for Tropical Medicine & Hygiene (FRSTMH), London, UK; a Fellow of the Faculty of Travel Medicine (FFTM) of the Royal College of Physicians and Surgeons of Glasgow (RCPSG), Glasgow, Scotland, UK; and a Fellow of the American College of Epidemiology (FACE), USA. He is also a candidate for Doctor in Parasitology (PhD), Universidad Central de Venezuela. He is a Doctor of Sciences honoris causa (HonDSc) from Universidad Privada Franz Tamayo (UniFranz), Cochabamba, Bolivia. Prof. Rodriguez-Morales is the President of the Travel Medicine Committee, Pan American ID Association, and the Vice President of the Colombian ID Association. He is a Senior Researcher of Colciencias (2017-2019), and a Professor at the Universidad Tecnológica de Pereira, Pereira, Risaralda, Colombia (H index=28). .

Editor of Volume 3:
Alfonso J. Rodriguez-Morales
Director of Research, Faculty of Health Sciences, Universidad Tecnológica de Pereira, Pereira, Risaralda, Colombia

Book Series Editor:
Shailendra K. Saxena
King George's Medical University

Scope of the Series

The series will give a most comprehensive overview of recent trends in various infectious diseases (as per the most recent Baltimore classification), as well as general concepts of infections, immunopathology, diagnosis, treatment, epidemiology and etiology to current clinical recommendations in management of infectious diseases, highlighting the ongoing issues, recent advances, with future directions in diagnostic approaches and therapeutic strategies. This book series will focus on various aspects and properties of infectious diseases whose deep understanding is very important for safeguarding human race from more loss of resources and economies due to pathogens.

Contents

Preface

Neglected tropical diseases (NTDs) is a diverse group of communicable diseases that prevail in tropical and subtropical conditions in 149 countries. NTDs affect more than one billion people and cost developing economies billions of dollars every year. According to the World Health Organization (WHO), NTDs mainly affect populations living in poverty, without adequate sanitation, and in close contact with infectious vectors, domestic animals, and livestock. Migration, as well as climate change and variability, are key factors in NTD prevalence (11-13). Therefore, NTDs deserve more study.

Recently, viruses transmitted by vectors (arboviruses) that affect not only people living in the tropics, but also travelers and migrating populations, have been causing epidemics. These viruses include Dengue, Chikungunya, Zika, Mayaro, and encephalitis viruses. These viruses emerge and reemerge in multiple regions of the world, as occurred in the Americas recently (2013-2017) with Chikungunya and Zika.

Keeping these issues in mind, this book includes different aspects of research and clinical topics related to relevant NTDs, including their implications for public health. This book has been organized in two sections: I. Vector-Borne Diseases; and, II. Zoonotic Diseases. Section I includes topics related to Dengue, Japanese Encephalitis, Chikungunya, and vector control. Section II includes experiences on Leprosy and Chagas Disease.

Commissioning of this book by IntechOpen was due, in part to my long commitment to vector-borne, zoonotic, and neglected tropical diseases, being involved as Co-Chair of the Working Group on Zoonoses of the International Society for Chemotherapy (WGZ-ISC), as well in Colombia at the Committee on Tropical Medicine, Zoonoses and Travel Medicine of the Colombian Association of Infectious Diseases (Asociación Colombiana de Infectología, ACIN) and more recently, as the Chair of the Colombian Collaborative Network of Research on Zika (Red Colombiana de Colaboración en Zika) (RECOLZIKA), since January 2016.

I have been involved in NTDs for the last two decades, including Leishmaniasis, Chagas Disease, and Dengue, and since 2014, Chikungunya and emerging arboviruses, such as Zika and Mayaro. After moving from Venezuela to Colombia in 2011, I have been involved in NTD research in Risaralda, such as Leishmaniasis (still prevalent in the area). Part of this work is a clear reflection of the work mission at the Research Group Infection Public Health and Infection (classified A1 by Colciencias) of the Faculty of Health Sciences of the Universidad Tecnológica de Pereira, directed by Dr. Guillermo Javier Lagos-Grisales, who is not just a partner, colleague, and friend, but also an extreme believer in our work in vector-borne and zoonotic diseases. I must also recognize the beginning of a significant collaboration after a meeting in Cartagena in 2013, during the

Colombian Congress of Infectious Diseases, where I met Dr. Wilmer Ernesto Villamil-Gómez, from Sincelejo, Sucre, Colombia, also part of the formerly known Committee of Zoonoses and Hemorrhagic Fevers of the Colombian Association of Infectious Diseases (Asociación Colombiana de Infectología, ACIN) (now called Committee of Zoonoses and Tropical Medicine), who became my most important collaborator on arboviruses, including Zika. In addition to this, since 2002 I have been involved in tropical medicine and travel medicine, participating in multiple studies on Chagas Disease, Leishmaniasis, and other tropical diseases. Currently in Colombia, we continue to study most of them, including in internally displaced populations.

Following the same philosophy as my eight previous books with IntechOpen (Current Topics in Tropical Medicine, Current Topics in Public Health, Current Topics in Echinococcosis, Current Topics in Chikungunya, Current Topics in Malaria, Current Topics in Giardiasis, Current Topics in Zika, Current Topics in Tropical Emerging Infectious Diseases and Travel Medicine this book does not intend to be an exhaustive compilation. This first edition has included multiple different topics and a wide geographical participation from many countries from different regions of the world. Its online availability, as well the possibility to upload the complete book or their chapters to personal websites and institution repositories, allows it to reach a wide. Continuing on the series of "Current Topics" books, we are planning to develop other projects such as "Current Topics in Zoonoses" and "Current Topics in Virology".

I would like to thank IntechOpen, and particularly to Andrea Koric (Commissioning Editor), for the opportunity to edit this interesting and important book, as well for her constant support.

I want to take the appropriate time and space to dedicate this book to my beloved family (Aurora, Alfonso José, Alejandro, and Andrea, the neurologist). Katterine, also I need to dedicate this book and further, to you. You arrived unexpectedly in my life to make it happier than ever. I love you with all my heart, my mind, and my soul.

Also, to my friends and my undergraduate and postgraduate students of health sciences in Colombia, Venezuela, and around Latin America. Thank you to my colleagues at the Working Group on Zoonoses, International Society for Chemotherapy, and the Committee on Zoonoses, Tropical Medicine and Travel Medicine (formerly Zoonoses and Haemorrhagic Fevers) of the ACIN and a large list of members of RECOLZIKA (www.RECOLZIKA.org). Special thanks again to my friend and colleague Dr. Guillermo J. Lagos-Grisales, MD, MPH. Members of our research group and incubator consist of young and enthusiastic medical students and some veterinary medical students as well as young medical doctors, who are pursuing significant improvements in the understanding of the epidemiology of zoonotic, vector-borne, parasitic, and infectious diseases in our country with international projection. 2019 has been a great year, very productive for this recognized group, which was classified in 2017 by the national agency of science, Colciencias, in the highest rank "A1", and then recognized again in 2019 with that rank, therefore positioning themselves as leaders in infectious diseases epidemiology research in the coffee-triangle region and in the country.

Finally, I hope our readers enjoy this publication as much as I did editing the chapters of Current Topics in Neglected Tropical Diseases.

Alfonso J. Rodriguez-Morales, MD, MSc, DTM&H, FRSTMH(Lon), FFTM RCPS(Glasg), FACE, PhD(c), Dr h c(HonDSc)
Professor,
Part-Time Faculty Instructor, Risk Factors (Epidemiology) (Coordinator),
Department of Community Medicine, School of Medicine,
Lecturer, Frontiers Research, Research IV,
School of Veterinary Medicine & Zootechnics,
Director of Research, Faculty of Health Sciences,
Universidad Tecnológica de Pereira,
Pereira, Risaralda, Colombia

Chair, Colombian Network of Research in Zika (RECOLZIKA)
Co-Chair, Working Group on Zoonoses,
International Society for Chemotherapy (ISC),
Vice President, Colombian Association of Infectious Diseases (ACIN),
Member of the Committee on Tropical Medicine,
Zoonoses and Travel Medicine, ACIN,
President, ACIN Chapter Coffee Triangle Region,
President, Committee on Travel Medicine,
Pan-American Association of Infectious Diseases,
Senior Researcher, Colciencias (2019-2021)

Section 1

Vector - Borne Diseases

Chapter 1

Persistent Barriers to Implementing Efficacious Mosquito Control Activities in the Continental United States: Insights from Vector Control Experts

Imelda K. Moise, Leo C. Zulu, Douglas O. Fuller and John C. Beier

Abstract

Many barriers undermine vector surveillance and control efforts in the United States. Experts warn that such barriers, including funding, threaten the capacity of public-health surveillance systems to detect emerging mosquito-borne disease and respond appropriately, timely and effectively. This chapter explores the status, barriers, and corrective strategies to effective mosquito surveillance and control in the US based on experiences and insights of the 35 interviewed representatives of diverse mosquito-control programs selected from 18 U.S. states. Although our interest is in mosquito-borne diseases, we focus on the 2016 Zika outbreak. For the most part, this chapter will outline issues relating to mosquito control and surveillance that have persistent among state, county and municipal programs as a result of insufficient and unreliable funding, inadequate trained personnel, poor facilities, and inadequate political support. At the community level, we will discuss issues that hinder mosquito control efforts including apathy and low public awareness, and provide examples of how mosquito control agencies have adapted to "readily" respond to changing vector-borne disease environments, demands and constrained funding.

Keywords: mosquito-borne diseases, Zika, barriers, mosquito control, United States

1. Introduction

The question of how ready United States (U.S.) public health officials are to prevent and control vector-borne disease transmission has received considerable attention since the first West Nile Virus (WNV) outbreak of 1999 in New York renewed by the recent Zika virus (ZIKV) outbreak. The first reported case of local ZIKV transmission through infected mosquitoes in the Continental United States was in Miami, Florida, in late July 2015. Although the global problem of mosquito-borne diseases (MBDs) is "as old as the pyramids" [1], it is a critical time to revisit mosquito control because despite significant gains in reducing the risk and incidence of some MBDs (particularly malaria); the world has seen a rise in the risk and incidence of other MBDs. This is particularly true for viruses transmitted via *Aedes* mosquitoes, such as *Chikungunya*, *Dengue* and ZIKV [2–4]. At the same time, it is nearly impossible to eliminate the local risk of transmission of exotic arbovirus once introduced to an area. Therefore, responding to exotic emerging arbovirus poses new challenges for mosquito control programs [5], as characterized below:

> *"The unpredictable nature and severity of vector-borne disease outbreaks demonstrates the urgent need for careful preparation and the incorporation of vector-control emergency-management activities into overall public health preparedness efforts"* [6].

Experts also worry that although prevention of MBDs is the best way forward and is substantially less costly than mosquito and disease control in response to a disease outbreak [7], MBD surveillance and control continued to be underfunded and to be the subject of budget cuts. In the 2011 U.S. fiscal year, a proposal was made to reduce funding for the Centers for Disease Control and Prevention (CDC)'s MBD program by $26.7 million [8]. The 2016 Congressional resistance and seven-month delay before approving former President Obama's request for emergency funding for ZIKV control [9] further illustrates such challenges. Such moves threaten the capacity of the existing public-health surveillance systems and response activities to deal with MBDs, such as the human WNV disease, Dengue and the ZIKV [10]. A national survey of the 50 state health departments reported a reduction in federal funding for mosquito surveillance of 61% between 2004 and 2012. This reduction resulted in non-tracking of active human cases of WNV in 22% of 56 jurisdictions (mosquito-control districts or territories), discontinued mosquito surveillance in 13%, reduced effort on mosquito trapping and testing in 70%, and reduction in WNV surveillance personnel by 38% [11, 12]. This does not bode well for the recent ZIKV outbreak in Florida and Texas, the serious birth defects it causes in babies, and the current lack limited planning to deal with it [13, 14]. Clinical tests for the ZIKV infection are of limited reliability and there is no vaccine to prevent ZIKV transmission directly from mosquitos or through the sexual transmission pathway. This makes surveillance and control of fundamental importance to prevent further ZIKV transmission and to prepare for dealing with other exotic arboviruses [15].

Maintaining sustainable systems for MBD surveillance can help define the nature and extent of the mosquito problem, provide a basis for evaluating the risk of transmission of MBDs, reduce the cost of responding to emerging vector-borne pathogens and ultimately gauge the efficacy of control activities [8]. While some research has been done on MBD control generically (though Hadler et al., [11, 12] as one exception), little has been done to explore variation in approaches, capacities and the quality of mosquito surveillance and control programs for emerging MBDs across the U.S., let alone from experiences and perceptions of mosquito-control Experts. Few studies have investigated the capacity to effectively surveil, prevent, and control arbovirus infections such as the ZIKV in the US.

In this chapter, inspired by the 2016 ZIKV outbreak in Florida, we use telephone interviews and qualitative research methods in understanding the diversity of current barriers and strategies to implementing efficacious mosquito surveillance and control in the Continental United States, particularly drawing on experiences and perspectives of active vector-control Experts. Insights from Experts can yield a range of locally relevant information that is difficult to obtain from traditional epidemiologic studies. Experts whose perspectives are included in this chapter include those working with state, county, municipal and other local mosquito-control programs or districts. Furthermore, we also provide variation in the

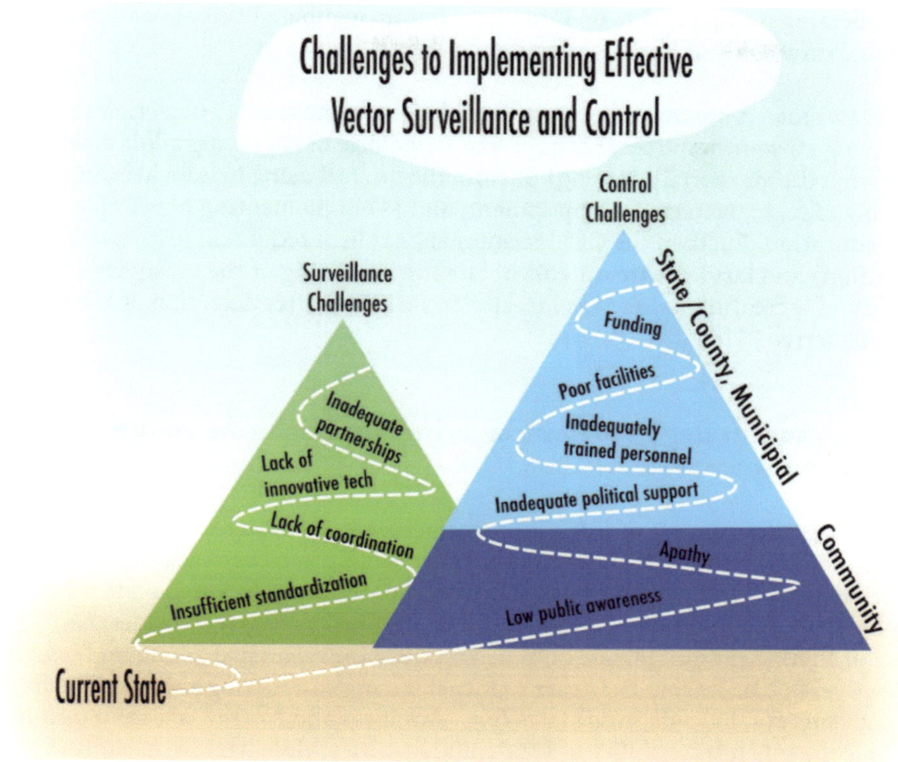

Figure 1.
Challenges that must be addressed before effective vector surveillance and control can be implemented according to the perspectives of 35 interviewed representatives of diverse mosquito-control programs selected from 18 U.S. states.

perceived capacities of state and local mosquito-control programs with different funding structures and state locations across the six US regions, to respond quickly and adequately to emerging MBD threats within the context of Integrated Vector Management (**Figure 1**).

2. Integrated vector management

Integrated vector management involves the optimum use of a mix of methods and resources for the efficient, cost-effective, ecologically sound and sustainable vector management (surveillance and control) in order to control vector-borne diseases. Surveillance of the *Aedes aegypti* and *Aedes albopictus* mosquitos that transmit the Dengue, Chikungunya, and ZIKV viruses generally involves:

1. Determining absence or presence of the vectors in a particular area

2. Identifying the main types of breeding containers for targeted control

3. Detailed mapping of larval sites for the vectors if found in the area

4. Collecting mosquito-population data and identifying density hotspots (high risk)

5. Monitoring impact of control efforts, and

6. Collecting mosquito data on infection rates in ongoing outbreaks and determine thresholds of human infection [14].

Effective mosquito-control programs traditionally include (1) detecting and monitoring mosquito sources; (2) applying larvicides; (3) applying adulticide treatments from the air (aerial spraying) or from the ground using handheld or more mechanized (e.g., from trucks) equipment; and (4) implementing outreach and public education. Further, the CDC recommends source reduction (e.g., container elimination) and larvicide treatments before the beginning of the mosquito season, and adulticide treatments, such as insecticide spraying, after detection of human arbovirus activity [14].

3. Barriers and strategies to implementing sustainable mosquito control and surveillance systems

Statewide mosquito surveys are an essential tool to monitor the presence, diversity, intensity and spatial distribution of mosquito vectors in a state. Responses showed that half (9) of the surveyed states had ever conducted a statewide mosquito-vector survey, and many of the rest had outdated surveys. The oldest conducted in 1940 (Arkansas) while only Arizona and Delaware had conducted one the previous year (2015). Only Delaware reported having conducting annual statewide mosquito surveys. In some rural states (e.g., Arkansas and North Dakota) mosquito control is the sole responsibility of local municipalities while in more urbanized states special mosquito control districts often complement local programs.

Responsibility and capacity for mosquito-vector surveillance and control varied across states. Knowledge about mosquitoes was greatest for mosquito species of concern to public health (e.g., *Aedes aegypti*, *Aedes albopictus*, and *Culex* species of mosquitoes). These species shaped the surveillance in most local programs. Asked if the ZIKV was an immediate public health concern in their state, respondents in sampled Southern States indicated that ZIKV was an enormous problem. Most respondents in surveyed Northern States indicated that locally transmitted ZIKV was not an immediate problem, mainly because the vectors are rare, absent, or another MBD (e.g., WNV) was more important:

> *ZIKV is not an issue in our state at all, as far as mosquito transmission because we do not have the mosquito Aedes aegypti. It has never been here and we certainly do not expect it to be here. Even the second vector, Aedes albopictus is extremely rare. WNV is much more serious here,* (Mosquito Control Contractor).

Others, while focusing on WNV control, indicated that it was only a matter of time before ZIKV carrying *Aedes aegypti or Aedes albopictus* arrives in their states, as this Mid-western respondent stated:

> *We are going to have a response on it but we are going to continue to work on WNV because WNV kills people in Illinois,* (Independent Mosquito Control Respondent).

3.1 Barriers to mosquito control

3.1.1 Inadequate and inconsistent funding

Mosquito-control efforts and their effectiveness vary greatly among control programs. The biggest factor perceived to determine effective mosquito surveillance and control programs and activities was the funding structure. Almost all the independent mosquito-control district respondents reported having dedicated, well-funded and stable mosquito control programs. The most common sources of funding for these self-funding or autonomous and semi-autonomous districts were local taxes (e.g., a small portion of property taxes and water bills) and revenues for contract work from private companies. On contrast, although respondents in dependent districts reported having a separate stable budget-line item for mosquito-control activities, their funding comes from county budgets and is therefore vulnerable to cuts where and when non-mosquito activities and programs have higher priority.

There was near consensus among Experts from state, county, municipal or other local programs that funding dedicated to mosquito-control activities was insufficient, unstable, and unpredictable. These programs were the most vulnerable to significant budget deficits and inconsistencies because they compete for funding with other departments and programs under tight municipal, county or County Boards of Commissioner budgets. Some interviewees felt that their agencies placed lower priority on mosquito-control activities. This forces them to be more reactive to outbreaks than proactive, an unlearnt lesson of the WNV outbreak with negative implications for program size, content, continuity and effectiveness in the context of the ZIKV outbreak:

> *...You have your director who is running the program but he has very little control over how money is spent. Therefore, when appropriated for mosquito control, but if another department is hurting in the budget arena, they can take some of mosquito control money,* (County Mosquito Control Respondent).

> *We have known even before the days of ZIKV, realizing the importance of mosquito surveillance. Again, sometimes it takes a crisis to make people respond,* (State Mosquito Control Respondent).

3.1.2 Institutional and logistical barriers

Institutional and logistical factors also impeded local vector surveillance and control programs, particularly state, municipal and county programs. Most Experts agreed that facilities and trained staff with requisite skills (e.g., in entomological skills) were insufficient. These shortages undermined essential activities such as effective specimen collection, vector identification, monitoring spatial mosquito distribution, MBD species present, number of cases in the locality, and the continuity of these activities. In a minority of cases, the lack of expertise can be extreme:

> *...A lot of them, they do not have even the expertise where the person who is responsible for the mosquito control is their City Maintenance Worker or their City Water Commissioner. Sometimes it is even the City Auditor. In the small communities, it is sometimes the garbage man* (State Mosquito Control Respondent).

Funding predictability and sustainability emerged as essential requirements to maintain programs and capacity to address emerging MBDs such as the ZIKV infection effectively. Respondents in cash-strapped programs generally attributes funding inconsistences to lack of or vacillating political will. There was consensus on the institutionally disruptive impacts of unreliable funding. These included laying off staff, scaling back surveillance and control activities such limiting mosquito-control activities to larviciding instead of the more targeted and effective adult mosquito-control applications, and suspending such activities altogether in some years. Respondent illustrates such impacts:

> *Once we get money out there and start funding vector control, then all of a sudden, it stops, then people think that we do not care anymore or that it was not the threat that we thought it was originally. ...long-term, level, stabilized funding from year to year is the only way to get a good vector control problem in to where we can actually mitigate the potential for disease transmission,* (County Mosquito Control Respondent).

The importance of continuity is such that while most respondents were skeptical that Congress would approve all or part of the federal emergency funding requested for ZIKV control by the Obama Administration in February 2016 in a timely manner, a small number paradoxically worried that some federal funding if provided would be unsustainable. They worried about building a technically and operationally costly surveillance and control program needed for arboviruses on a shaky foundation of federal funding that they considered particularly vulnerable to budget cuts:

> *We go through a few blank years with limited programs in place because we do not have funding to move forward with it. Then ZIKV hits and it becomes a national concern again and my biggest fear is the Federal Government will be nice enough to pass the budget and get money out but that funding isn't sustainable,* (County Mosquito Control Respondent).

> *I am afraid we'll get a good program in place like the one we did with WNV and have surveillance and outreach and really get some abatement going, then all of a sudden the funding dries up and you're stuck again with the need to do something without the capability of doing something,* (State Mosquito Control Respondent).

Ultimately, funding unpredictability undercuts the ability to be proactive, a critical component of MBD control:

> *Once a disease has entered and gotten hold, it's much more difficult to eliminate or control that disease, as opposed to being proactive, monitoring the situation and if a threat is identified, to establish some sort of game plan to be able to control the disease,* (Independent Mosquito Control Respondent).

Some states have sought to balance quality surveillance and cost under tight budgets. Thus, Arkansas traps for the presence/absence of mosquitoes along (both side) of county boundaries. This provides an even geographic spread for vector sampling within a limited area while providing the opportunity to share costs among bordering counties. Many programs focus surveillance on larvae because they know likely breeding sites, such as water containers for *Aedes aegypti,* and bias adult surveillance to areas that have had high *Aedes aegypti* densities in the past.

Another major institutional challenge was inadequate coordination across program service areas. As a mosquito control contractor noted, "there are always mosquitoes flying from outside of your control area," and sometimes beyond their geographic range. Most respondents indicated that this cross-boundary mosquito mobility challenged their response since all surveyed programs (except in Arkansas) limited their activities within their county, township, or other jurisdictional boundaries. Further, differences in resource availability, capacity, methods and priority of vector control across control jurisdictions results in fragmented mosquito surveillance and control and creates gaps in coverage, which undermine the ability of mosquito-control programs to mitigate the risk of MBD transmission across landscapes.

3.1.3 Low public awareness and apathy on mosquito efforts

Most respondents decried apathy (lack of interest or concern), low public awareness of the need and nature of mosquito control, and low political will. This undermined community co-operation in mosquito surveillance and control, including limiting access to private property for trap placement, and participation in mosquito control at the household level (e.g., clearing containers). Further, many respondents cited resistance to chemical use for mosquito abatement among some community members based on environmental concerns, especially adverse non-target impacts, as well as on philosophical opposition to chemicals. They were particularly wary of such worldviews and attitudes because they can erode community trust and co-operation, and undermine control efforts:

> *...we have many people who are philosophically opposed to what we do and they are misinformed, they expose themselves to all sorts of misinformation from various advocacy groups who are anti-pesticides,* (Mosquito Control Contractor).

Many respondents indicated that they had come a long way in balancing public health and environmental concerns. This includes using the most environmentally friendly control chemicals. They also highlighted apathy and lack of knowledge among the public as a major barrier. Nearly all underscored public education as necessary to enhance mosquito control through individual behavior change and to gain community support for programs (including improved budgets and equipment). Many admitted that previous public-education efforts had been inadequate, and often ineffective to effect positive behavioral change. Still, it was clear that Experts considered public education, community engagement, outreach, and media attention important strategies to overcome apathy and mitigate negative perceptions of mosquito control.

Enhanced and more effective public education emerged as an important strategy to address some of the some of the barriers. Respondents recognized the role of federal agencies (e.g., CDC) and states in public education and information dissemination, particularly during disease outbreaks. However, many preferred approaches that involved person-to-person contact, particularly door-to-door visits and school outreach, for their effectiveness in both getting cooperation and participation, and in passing on the message to others in the community. Some respondents indicated that neighborhood residents who actually experience mosquito management efforts were more likely to support vector and pest control programs. Outreach and integration of vector prevention and surveillance in schools is favored as a powerful tool to reach parents through school-going children while also preparing a future generation of informed leaders:

> *We actually have an educational outreach person who works in our biology department and she goes to schools and works with the science teachers ...educating kids on mosquitoes and all aspects of their breeding and how to control them,* (State Mosquito Control Respondent).

3.2 Barriers to mosquito surveillance

3.2.1 Lack of standards on sampling and of evaluation of impacts of sub-optimal trap placement on MBD-risk assessment

Interviews revealed wide variation in mosquito-surveillance practices. Beyond virtual consensus that integrated vector management (IVM) is the ideal approach, there were no agreed standards on practices, including accuracy criteria for estimates. There was wide variation in the type, number, sampling protocol, spacing and frequency of mosquito-trap placement across programs. Location of traps was based on diverse and sometimes subjective factors heavily dependent on local contingencies such as resource availability, local Expert knowledge, and convenience. Factors included the practical need to locate traps away from public view to prevent human disturbance and vandalism (deliberate destruction) and accessibility—many practitioners placed traps in public spaces (parks, natural areas) and on properties of willing residents. While laws on access to private property for mosquito abatement varied across states, respondents often negotiated with individual residents for access and permission to place traps thereon. The type of mosquito trap used and the need to avoid vandalism or theft also mattered. Traps that require electricity, such as the New Jersey light traps, commonly used for *Aedes aegypti* and *Aedes albopictus,* are placed close to built-up areas with electricity supply. There was also a bias toward areas already known to have high mosquito densities. The following quotes illustrate some of the locally specific and sometimes-subjective factors that determined sampling particularly trap placements:

> *You want to place it somewhere where you are going to find mosquitos but it comes down to where I can hang it. We have our ideal of where we want to set it, and then it is rather where we can set it,* (Independent Mosquito Control Respondent).

> *You try to cover the area the best you can, but, you know, just depends on what your limitations are. However, for an everyday surveillance, it would not be a good idea just to go to a specific neighborhood and put a bunch of traps out,* (Dependent Mosquito Control Respondent).

> *We sometimes do not' have control over where those traps are placed when there is a volunteer setting traps,* (State Mosquito Control Respondent).

The problems of inadequate and unpredictable funding undermining mosquito control also afflict surveillance. Respondents noted that limited resources (funding, trained staff and others) often promote convenience sampling rather than optimal IVM practice. While some of the resulting inconsistencies are expected to vary due to local and regional variation in vector ecology and MBD transmission dynamics, they undermine cross-jurisdiction coordination and effective surveillance; many respondents noted the need for some standardization.

Reliability of mosquito-surveillance practices is important to guide sound decision-making on control interventions such as source reduction, larvicide treatment and adult reductions (e.g., adulticide). Some respondents admitted that their programs conducted little mosquito testing. A state mosquito-control Expert indicated that some programs conducted testing only when they note unusually high numbers of mosquitoes. While many small communities will use test results to trigger local vector control, "some of them don't even look at the data." Most Experts indicated that they used thresholds (e.g., mosquito larvae, pupal or adult density) derived from mosquito-surveillance data as triggers for fogging or spraying. The thresholds, nevertheless, appeared not standardized and varied greatly by program and species, and some were vague:

> *There is a threshold set that if the mosquito traps show higher than that—or we will send people out and if they report that the landing rate count is at a certain number, we will send planes out,* (Independent Mosquito Control Respondent).

> *In response to Culex, our action thresholds are 50 females or more. As far as Aedes aegypti, and based on work that we did last year, we came up with a numerical threshold of 50 or more females per trap. .... if any of the Aedes aegypti test positive for our arboviruses, then we will go ahead and fog too,* (County Mosquito Control Respondent).

Experts revealed common concerns that the current work environment was reactive rather than proactive and preventive. Many respondents decried the narrow focus on outbreaks of high profile MBDs—the so-called disease *du jour* or disease of the day, e.g., ZIKV, Dengue, and WNV—or on responding to extreme events such as hurricanes or flooding. Both tend to be geographically limited in scope. Many complained that this reactive approach undermined surveillance efforts and their capacity to detect, anticipate and respond to emerging MBDs instead of always playing catch-up:

> *Surveillance is important. Every couple of years, some mosquito disease captures the headlines. Today it is ZIKV; a couple years ago, it was Chikungunya and a couple years before that was West Nile Virus, which means a few years from now, something else will happen,* (Mosquito Control Contractor).

3.2.2 Coordination across mosquito control jurisdictions

Conversations affirmed the general view that at the local scale of operation below the state level the better for surveillance and control because such districts were better able to respond to the high level of variability in vector ecology and social and institutional contexts. With better and stable funding, independent mosquito districts maximized local-scale advantages. Respondents nevertheless highlighted the need for enhanced cross-jurisdiction coordination and some level of standardization of best practices for consistent mosquito surveillance within and across jurisdictions. Some state agencies played this cross-jurisdiction coordination role functionally, administratively or in a regulatory capacity, drawing on broad federal guidelines provided by the CDC and the Environmental Protection Agency. For example, respondents in Florida indicated that the Florida's Department of Agriculture and Consumer Services has Spot Teams that fill surveillance and control gaps by covering areas that have no funding or staff by using contractors or nearby programs, often on a cost-recovery basis in the case of disease control.

Florida also provides a commendable model for statewide coordination among mosquito-control Experts. A non-profit association, the Florida Mosquito Control Association (FMCA) was formed in1922 to promote the interests, exchange information and coordinate the activities members drawn from diverse mosquito-control programs. Coordination includes standardization of practice, information exchange, and professional training and certification. A representative explained FMCA origins and significance:

> *...there was a need for exchange of information and coordination throughout the state. ...to help coordinate and get information so that something that is found or discovered is shared with the rest of the State of Florida,* (FMCA Representative).

3.2.3 Partnerships are important

Almost all program respondents reported formal and informal partnerships with other relevant agencies working at different scales—local, county, state, and federal. In addition to drawing overall guidance from the CDC, most respondents cited the Environmental Protection Agency (EPA) as a federal partner. Local partners included the Department of Environmental Quality (DEQ), county health departments, Department of Agriculture and other government and county departments, universities, and other nearby mosquito-control districts, including local communities. Several respondents, particularly from resource-constrained programs, indicated that such partnerships allowed their programs to reduce or externalize some operational costs. Some gained access to external resources through formal contracts, memoranda of understanding (e.g., California), grants, collaboration with other agencies, community volunteers, and local schools. Many programs often used these partnerships to fill skill gaps with external expertise. Some programs extended their available resources though cost savings, use of private contractors, and provision of incentives including grants. The quotes below illustrate such collaboration:

> *They recruit anywhere from eighty to a hundred...We try to have at least one in every county...These are New Jersey traps. The people who are doing this collection, they are volunteering. Every week they will take their... light trap and mail it* (State Mosquito Surveillance Respondent).

> *We have a few contracts with county health departments to do mosquito control, usually surveillance. .... mostly, we work informally,* (Mosquito Control Contractor).

3.3 Future prospects for mosquito surveillance and control

In addition to the barriers identifies to effective mosquito surveillance and control in the context of the ZIKV outbreak, the research also revealed promising measures that can be taken to improve the situation. On funding barriers, findings affirmed the importance of increased funding. Given the nature of mosquito surveillance and control, and the consequent need for long-term investment, however, the predictability and sustenance of funding were even more important. The disruptive adverse impacts of reduced and inconsistent funding also illustrated in other studies, including stoppage of tracking of tracking of human cases of WNV, and reductions in mosquito trapping, testing and surveillance and personnel [10, 11], threaten effective surveillance, and early detection and prevention of MBD transmission, including for the ZIKV. This also includes inconsistent mosquito data from insufficient trap locations that undermine assessment of the risk of human exposure to the vector and MBDs [14, 16]. However, recent increases in funding for interventions and research offer new hope, so long as such funding is sustained particularly at municipal, county and state programs. Such funding includes $1.1 billion in emergency federal funding for ZIKV response (approved in September 2016), CDC funding of the establishment of four MBD s regional Centers of Excellence in the US (approved in December 2016), and state-level (Florida State funding of $25 million for the development of a ZIKV vaccine. Some gains can also be made in creative forms of financing and increases in efficiency in mosquito surveillance and control activities. **Table 1** presents the identified barriers and strategies to implementing sustainable mosquito control and surveillance systems in the US. Emerging ideas included more dependence on local (tax) funding sources as independent control districts, mosquito sampling along county boundaries to share and reduce costs (e.g., Kansas State), cross-jurisdiction collaboration and cost sharing, and the use of citizen science to enhance data collection.

In response to the challenge of lack of inconsistencies in mosquito surveillance techniques, the need for some degree of standardization in sampling protocols while accommodating vector spatial variability has also been noted in other studies.

Barriers	
Inadequate and inconsistent funding (mainly for state, county and municipal programs).	Policies focused on sustaining funding statewide mosquito surveillance and control capabilities.
	Developing partnerships for cost sharing and community training for participation in mosquito trapping, testing and prevention.
Lack of political will and support.	Enhanced public education—raise awareness and concern, influence politicians.
Complex trans-boundary mosquito risks and limited cross-boundary coordination.	Enhanced collaborative arrangements and cooperation across mosquito districts, e.g., skill sharing, contracts, memoranda of understanding, voluntarism.
Limited capacity and specially trained personnel.	Hire skilled personnel and train existing ones on needed skills.
	Use innovative technologies, e.g., smart traps.
	Statewide or regional Experts for mosquito programs and activities.
Philosophical and environmental belief barriers to mosquito control.	IVM—innovative mix of synergistic methods, e.g., environmentally friendly insecticides and application technologies, biological control, habitat reduction.
	More and effective public education and communication with stakeholders.
Legal abatement obstacles to timely response.	Promoting persuasive person-person community outreach to gain voluntary access.
Lack of standardization and inconsistent mosquito data from few trap locations and select locations	Develop standard surveillance methods for particular a subset of conditions, and quality control mechanisms.
	New research on vector biology, control methods and responsiveness to MBDs.
	Adequately funded and consistent surveillance for predicting and reducing human infection.

Table 1.
Barriers and strategies to implementing sustainable mosquito control and surveillance systems.

To be sure, some variability is expected, particularly in *mosquito-control* approaches and practices (e.g., in scope, prioritization, technical methods, etc.) given their need to adapt to geographic variation in vector ecology, MBD transmission dynamics, and socio-institutional conditions. However, for surveillance, Bowman et al., [22] also call for "standardized sampling protocols that adequately consider dengue spatial heterogeneity." Research on mosquito-vector sampling and its impacts on the accuracy of human risk assessment remains relatively limited [17, 18]. Some common mosquito indices are sensitive to sampling differences [18] and others are poorly statistically correlated to the actual risk of disease [17], compounding negative impacts of such inconsistencies. Efforts by the CDC to provide generic guidelines in the USA [13] and the World Health Organization (WHO) to do the same globally [19], and other isolated studies offer a starting point for standardization. One study in Cairns, Australia recommended a sampling intensity of one BG-Sentinel trap for an area of 150 by 150 m (two or three traps for three housing blocks) to monitor *Aedes aegypti,* given the limited spatial dispersal (as little as 78–200 m in some studies) of this container-breeding species [18]. Modern spatially explicit technologies, particularly remote sensing analysis and Geographic Information Systems (GIS), expand the sets of tools for mosquito surveillance at landscape scales. Thus, the Random sampling of trapping locations for *Aedes aegypti* in urban areas based on Geographic Information Systems and satellite imagery has been shown to improve the accuracy of entomological indices compared to those derived through the common biased method of selecting locations or houses that are known to have high vector densities [20].

There are also promising technological advances in mosquito control, including the introduction of biological control and low-cost, eco-friendly pesticides mosquito vectors and safeguard the environment and the public [19]. Recent (November 2016) FDA approval of field trials involving the release of genetically modified (GM) mosquitoes into the wild to control ZIKV and Zengue-carrying mosquitoes for in the Florida Keys, Florida, could increase the number of successful cases of biological control using GMO mosquitoes beyond Brazil and China. Non-GM mosquitoes infected with naturally occurring Wolbachia bacteria also offer early promise as a biological pesticide and have been field-tested in at least three US states against *Aedes albopictus*, and in Clovis city, Fresco County, California (2016) against male *Aedes aegypti* mosquitoes [21]. Gene editing using the CRISPR-Cas9 system facilitates the genetic engineering of mosquitoes to make them infertile or repel pathogens [22]. The use of organic or green-synthesized pesticides is also advancing the quest for inexpensive, nontoxic and eco-friendly methods for killing particular species of mosquitoes or their larvae and pupae. Examples include the use of green-synthesized pesticides, such as silver nanoparticles (AgNP) produced from seaweed (*Hypnea musciformis*) to kill the larvae and pupae of the vector *Aedes aegypti* alone [23] or in combination with mosquito-predator Asian bulldog tadpoles [24]. Other plants have also been tested, such as *Zornia diphylla* leaves against *Anopheles subpictus,* the dengue vector *Aedes albopictus* and the Japanese encephalitis vector Culex tritaeniorhynchus [25] (and the shoofly plant, *Nicandra physalodes, as a botanical* larvicidal *extract to control Anopheles stephensi*, *Aedes aegypti* (dengue vector), and *Culex quinquefasciatus* (filariasis vector) [26]. Although many of these technological advances are still some years before they can be approved for field application [19], more operational or implementation research is needed to further demonstrate their effectiveness in both mosquito control and cost under particularly settings, in order to accelerate their approval and wider use.

Our findings show that the low hanging fruit in improved mosquito-vector surveillance and control lie in improving the institutional capacity of the relevant mosquito-control agencies at local, county, state, and federal scales, and building/strengthening creative partnerships among researchers, mosquito-control Experts and jurisdictions, local communities, schools, and the public at large. Benefits of partnerships fell into four categories: (1) sharing resources and reducing operational costs; (2) reducing apathy and enhancing individual responsibility in household mosquito-control efforts, particularly through person-to-person contact (including citizen science in mosquito trapping and other data collection); (3) strengthening community support to enhance political will and support for more and stable funding; and (4) more effective and sustainable mosquito control across service boundaries. In addition, more effective public education strategies were also crucial, including those involving human contact and the use of volunteers and students in data collection and other mosquito-surveillance tasks under the label of citizen science.

4. Conclusion

While some of the barriers identified in this study are consistent with those identified previously, for instance in regard to WNV outbreaks, their persistence is worrisome. These inadequate surveillance and insufficient, reactive funding that prioritizes responses to the disease *du jour*, and vacillating political will First, funding barriers were acutely import for municipal, county and state mosquito programs. Independent and dependent taxing mosquito districts reported better funding and smoother operations. Second, continuity of funding emerged critical for effective IVM. Disruptions in funding interrupted critical surveillance or control efforts and institutional arrangements and partnerships that take time to build and are hard to replace and restart, threatening the capacity of programs to detect, prevent and control MBD outbreaks.

Another emerging challenge from Experts' perspectives was relatively high variability in *mosquito-surveillance* methods and practices, insufficient standardization and quality control. The lack of standardization can undermine the reliability of entomological indices of mosquito presence or abundance and thresholds derived from the disparate surveillance methods, and assessments of MBD transmission, and ensuing responses. In particular, disparities in practice on mosquito-vector sampling (method, size and representativeness) was a concern because its impacts on common mosquito indices and ultimately on the accuracy of human risk assessment was understudied and often unknown. A degree of standardization is needed to enhance scientific rigor and consistency in mosquito surveillance over space and time. Modern spatially explicit technologies particularly remote sensing analysis and GIS offer promising tools for sampling standardization and surveillance across scales.

Findings also revealed instances of, and further need for, creativity and accommodation among mosquito-control Experts under resource-strained conditions and competing interests that can provide insights for further research and development of best practice for particular settings. Examples include cost-effective and methodologically sound mosquito sampling and MBD risk assessments, adjusting the timing or spatial targeting of insecticide application to meet methodological and special-interest needs (e.g., to minimize harm to bees and maintain good relations with beekeepers); or skipping of particular houses whose owners do not want truck-fogging. Findings further revealed the need to determine the minimum set of surveillance services needed given the tight funding conditions of state, county and municipal programs.

Building effective partnerships among public, private and academic/research institutions, local communities and schools emerged as an important strategy among most mosquito-control Experts. An outstanding challenge was finding effective ways to address opposition to the use of pesticides in mosquito control among local communities. Creative and sustained methods to educate the public on the dangers and benefits of MBD and mosquitos are also needed.

Looking ahead, perspectives of Experts from this exploratory study reveal that increased and reliable funding is a priority to mitigate many of the barriers, ensure effective surveillance and early detection and prevention of MBD transmission at municipal, county or local, and state levels. Recent new funding for responding to the 2016/16 ZIKV outbreak and for research by the US Congress and the CDC at federal level, as well as at state level for at-risk states such as Florida, are promising developments. However, the long-term value lies in their ability to enhance the capacity, cost-effectiveness, and sustainability of programs at multiple scales.

Further introduction into integrated pest management approaches of biological control and low-cost, eco-friendly pesticides hold considerable promise for the mosquitoes and MBD control in the near future while safeguarding the environment and public health broadly. Examples include the release of genetically modified (GM) mosquitoes into the wild to control ZIKV and Dengue-carrying mosquitoes under FDA-approved field-testing in the Florida Keys, Florida, USA. Non-GM mosquitoes infected with naturally occurring *Wolbachia* bacteria also offer early promise as a biological pesticide (in at least three US states) against *Aedes albopictus and Aedes aegypti*. Research is also advancing on organic or green-synthesized pesticides as inexpensive, nontoxic and eco-friendly methods for killing particular species of mosquitoes or their larvae and pupae.

While this study exploratory, qualitative study of is not meant to be statistically representative or generalizable to the entire U.S. of all settings, it offers a wide range of perspectives and insights from mosquito-control Experts on issues including the nature and range of barriers and opportunities for mosquito-vector control in Continental United States. More detailed empirical analysis in selected states, which have had recent outbreaks or are at high risk of ZIKV, such as Florida, Texas and Louisiana, is the next step in terms of research.

Acknowledgements

We thank all the 35 mosquito Experts who participated in the interviews and the research assistants who helped interview them. This publication was supported by Cooperative Agreement Number U01CK000510, funded by the Centers for Disease Control and Prevention. Its contents are solely the responsibility of the authors and do not necessarily represent the official views of the Centers for Disease Control and Prevention or the Department of Health and Human Services.

Conflict of interest

The authors declare no conflict of interest.

Abbreviations

AgNP	silver nanoparticles
CDC	Centers for Disease Control
DEQ	Department of Environmental Quality
EPA	Environmental Protection Agency
FDA	Food and Drug Administration
FMCA	Florida Mosquito Control Association
GIS	geographic information system
GM	genetically modified
GMO	genetically modified organism
IVM	integrated vector management
MBD	mosquito-borne diseases
WHO	World Health Organization
WNV	West Nile virus
ZIKV	Zika virus

Author details

Imelda K. Moise[1,3]*, Leo C. Zulu[2], Douglas O. Fuller[1] and John C. Beier[3]

1 Department of Geography and Regional Studies, College of Arts and Sciences, University of Miami, USA

2 Department of Geography, Environment and Spatial Sciences, Michigan State University, USA

3 Department of Public Health Sciences, Miller School of Medicine, University of Miami, USA

*Address all correspondence to: moise@miami.edu

References

[1] Hanem FK. Introductory chapter: Back to the future—Solutions for parasitic problems as old as the pyramids, natural remedies in the fight against parasites. In: Khater DH, editor. Natural Remedies in the Fight Against Parasites. Rijeka, Croatia: InTech; 2017

[2] Slutsker L, Kachur SP. It is time to rethink tactics in the fight against malaria. Malaria Journal. 2013;**12**:140. DOI: 10.1186/1475-2875-12-140

[3] Cauchemez S, Ledrans M, Poletto C, Quenel P, de Valk H, Colizza V, et al. Local and regional spread of chikungunya fever in the Americas. Euro Surveillance. 2014;**19**:20854

[4] Fauci AS, Morens DM. Zika virus in the Americas—Yet another arbovirus threat. New England Journal of Medicine. 2016;**374**:601-604

[5] Hemingway J. The role of vector control in stopping the transmission of malaria: Threats and opportunities. Philosophical Transactions of the Royal Society of London. Series B, Biological Sciences. 2014;**369**:20130431

[6] McKenna M. Disorganized mosquito control will make US vulnerable to Zika. Germination. 2016. Available from: http://phenomena.nationalgeographic.com/2016/02/29/zika-mosquito-control/

[7] ASTHO. Public Health Confronts the Mosquito: Developing Sustainable State and Local Mosquito Control Programs. Washington, DC: ASTHO; 2005

[8] Vazquez-Prokopec GM, Chaves LF, Ritchie SA, Davis J, Kitron U. Unforeseen costs of cutting mosquito surveillance budgets. PLoS Neglected Tropical Diseases. 2010;**4**:e858

[9] STAT. Congress Approves $1.1 Billion in Zika Funding. 2016

[10] Couzin-Frankel J. Infectious diseases. Fears of lax surveillance if CDC program cut. Science. 2010;**328**:1088

[11] Hadler JL, Patel D, Nasci RS, Petersen LR, Hughes JM, Bradley K, et al. Assessment of arbovirus surveillance 13 years after introduction of West Nile virus, United States. Emerging Infectious Diseases. 2015;**21**:1159-1166

[12] Hadler JL, Patel D, Bradley K, Hughes JM, Blackmore C, Etkind P, et al. National capacity for surveillance, prevention, and control of West Nile virus and other arbovirus infections—United States, 2004 and 2012. MMWR. Morbidity and Mortality Weekly Report. 2014;**63**:281-284

[13] Shanker D. Zika Is here, and America has no plan to fight it. Bloomberg. 2016

[14] CDC. Surveillance and Control of *Aedes aegypti* and *Aedes albopictus* in the United States. 2016. Available from: http://www.cdc.gov/chikungunya/resources/vector-control.html

[15] Berkelman RL, Bryan RT, Osterholm MT, LeDuc JW, Hughes JM. Infectious disease surveillance: A crumbling foundation. Science. 1994;**264**:368-370

[16] Yoo E, Chen D, Russel C. West Nile Virus Mosquito Abundance Modeling Using Nonstationary Spatiotemporal Geostatistics. In: Chen D, Moulin B, Wu J, editors. Analyzing and Modeling Spatial and Temporal Dynamics of Infectious Diseases. 2015. DOI: 10.1002/9781118630013.ch14

[17] Bowman LR, Donegan S, McCall PJ. Is dengue vector control deficient in effectiveness or evidence? Systematic review and meta-analysis.

PLoS Neglected Tropical Diseases. 2016;**10**:e0004551

[18] Azil AH, Bruce D, Williams CR. Determining the spatial autocorrelation of dengue vector populations: Influences of mosquito sampling method, covariables, and vector control. Journal of Vector Ecology. 2014;**39**:153-163

[19] Fernandes JN, Moise IK, Maranto GL, Beier JC. Revamping mosquito-borne disease control to tackle future threats. Trends in Parasitology. 2018: S1471-4922(18)30008-4 DOI: 10.1016/j.pt.2018.01.005

[20] Troyo A, Fuller DO, Calderón-Arguedas O, Beier JC. A geographical sampling method for surveys of mosquito larvae in an urban area using high-resolution satellite imagery. Journal of Vector Ecology. 2008;**33**:1-7

[21] Zhang S. A California city is fending off Zika by releasing 40,000 mosquitoes every week. Science. 2016

[22] Hammond A, Galizi R, Kyrou K, Simoni A, Siniscalchi C, Katsanos D, et al. A CRISPR-Cas9 gene drive system targeting female reproduction in the malaria mosquito vector *Anopheles gambiae*. Nature Biotechnology. 2015;**34**:78

[23] Roni M, Murugan K, Panneerselvam C, Subramaniam J, Nicoletti M, Madhiyazhagan P, et al. Characterization and biotoxicity of *Hypnea musciformis*-synthesized silver nanoparticles as potential eco-friendly control tool against *Aedes aegypti* and *Plutella xylostella*. Ecotoxicology and Environmental Safety. 2015;**121**:31-38

[24] Murugan K, Priyanka V, Dinesh D, Madhiyazhagan P, Panneerselvam C, Subramaniam J, et al. Predation by Asian bullfrog tadpoles, *Hoplobatrachus tigerinus*, against the dengue vector, *Aedes aegypti*, in an aquatic environment treated with mosquitocidal nanoparticles. Parasitology Research. 2015;**114**(10):3601

[25] Govindarajan M, Rajeswary M, Muthukumaran U, Hoti SL, Khater HF, Benelli G. Single-step biosynthesis and characterization of silver nanoparticles using *Zornia diphylla* leaves: A potent eco-friendly tool against malaria and arbovirus vectors. Journal of Photochemistry and Photobiology B: Biology. 2016;**161**:482-489

[26] Govindarajan M, Khater HF, Panneerselvam C, Benelli G. One-pot fabrication of silver nanocrystals using *Nicandra physalodes*: A novel route for mosquito vector control with moderate toxicity on non-target water bugs. Research in Veterinary Science. 2016;**107**:95-101

Chapter 2

The Global Distribution and Burden of Dengue and Japanese Encephalitis Co-Infection in Acute Encephalitis Syndrome

Shailendra K. Saxena, Swatantra Kumar, Vimal K. Maurya and Madan L.B. Bhatt

Abstract

Dengue is widespread throughout the tropics globally in more than hundred countries and coincides with various climatic factors for co-infection with other flaviviral infections of the central nervous system (CNS). Dengue and Japanese encephalitis virus co-infection are highly prevalent, with diagnosis dilemma including significant mortality and morbidity in Southeast Asia. Both dengue and Japanese encephalitis transmissions intensify during the rainy season, during which the vector population increases. CNS involvement during dengue and Japanese encephalitis co-infection-associated acute encephalitis syndrome (AES) is still poorly understood, and therefore, there is a desperate need to understand the etiology, therapeutics, clinical management, and prevention of these tropically neglected diseases. AES can be differentiated from other etiologies of encephalopathy through considering its essential features: sudden onset of fever, cerebrospinal fluid (CSF) comprising inflammatory cells, magnetic resonance imaging (MRI)-based confirmation, and presence of pathogen or pathogen-specific antibodies. Complementary and alternative medicine is progressively being used globally and can be effective for the overall management of this co-infection.

Keywords: dengue, Japanese encephalitis, co-infection, encephalitis, acute encephalitis syndrome (AES), differential diagnosis, treatment, management, prevention, complementary and alternative medicine

1. Introduction

Neglected tropical diseases (NTDs) are the diverse group of communicable diseases which exist in tropical and subtropical settings affecting more than one billion people worldwide [1]. Populations inhabiting places with poor sanitation are in close contact with infected vectors, and domestic animals are principally affected. Arthropod-borne or arboviruses such as dengue, Zika, and Chikungunya have been recently included in the list of NTDs by the World Health Organization [2].

Human infection of flavivirus may cause severe clinical manifestations and can be broadly subdivided into two groups as neurological diseases caused by Japanese encephalitis virus (JEV), West Nile virus, and Zika virus (ZIKV) and hemorrhagic and viscerotropic diseases caused by dengue virus (DENV), ZIKV, and yellow fever virus (YFV) [3]. More than half of the global population is now at the risk of getting flavivirus infections where the majority of areas are endemic for more than one flaviviruses which results in the phenomenon of co-infection [4]. The worldwide incident of dengue has extensively grown in few decades [5]. Majority of the dengue cases are asymptomatic, and therefore, it is hard to anticipate the accurate burden of the disease. The rise in number of cases from 2.2 million in the year 2010 to 3.34 million cases in 2016 suggests the sharp increase in the disease burden. The 2016 year is characterized as the largest outbreak for dengue where 2.38 million cases were reported from the region of the Americas where 1.5 million cases were contributed by Brazil alone. Currently 3.9 billion in 128 countries people are at risk of DENV infection [6]. Unlike dengue, Japanese encephalitis (JE) is confined to Southeast Asia and Western Pacific regions. Approximately 68,000 clinical cases of JE are reported annually with 13,000 to 24,000 deaths. Currently more than 3 billion in 24 countries are at risk of JEV infection [7]. The epidemiology of dengue and JE has been depicted in **Figure 1**.

DENV and JEV belongs to the *Flaviviridae* family, which consists of more than 70 viruses, comprising of single-stranded positive-sense RNA genome protected by envelope protein [8]. Viruses from this family belong to the genus *Flavivirus*, which are transmitted by mosquitoes or ticks and are characterized as arthropod-borne infections. The transmission cycle of *Flavivirus* involves animals including human which are considered to be the dead-end hosts [9]. Hematophagous mosquitoes are the transmission vector for these diseases. *Aedes albopictus* and *Aedes aegypti* mosquitoes are known to transmit the dengue virus, whereas *Culex tritaeniorhynchus* is predominantly involve in the transmission of JEV [10]. These viruses have been shown to be transmitted via transplacental route as well [11].

Pathogen-associated acute encephalitis syndrome (PA-AES) may result from diverse pathogenic infections including DENV and JEV. PA-AES shows a wide range of symptoms including headache, vomiting and severe illness, reduced consciousness, altered sensorium, convulsions, and tremors [12]. Flaviviruses share substantial sequence similarities to stimulate sero-cross-reactivity which results in the antibody-dependent enhancement (ADE) of infection with other flaviviruses [13].

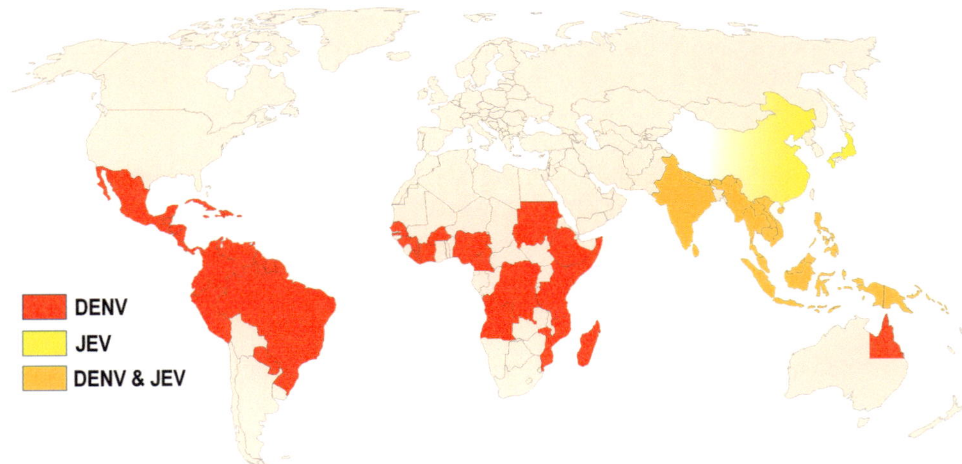

Figure 1.
Dengue and Japanese encephalitis epidemiology. The worldwide epidemiology of dengue and Japanese encephalitis has been depicted in this map. More than 100 countries are endemic for dengue where America, Western Pacific regions, and Southeast Asia are mostly affected. The Japanese encephalitis is confined to mostly in Southeast Asia and Western Pacific regions which include approximately 24 countries. The dengue-affected regions are highlighted in red color, JE-affected regions are highlighted in yellow color, and regions where both viruses are circulating have been highlighted in orange color.

Outbreaks of DENV co-infection are predominantly associated with the JEV endemic area or areas of JE immunization [14]. Although DENV-induced encephalitis is rare, the co-infection may increase the severity of encephalitis. DENV infection causes dengue hemorrhagic fever (DHF), whereas JEV infection may result in neurological complications [15]. Intermittently, DENV has been reported to cause encephalitis, and JEV infection may cause extraneural hemorrhage [16, 17]. However, this may not be the case in co-infection with both the flaviviruses. Simultaneous detection of both the viruses is not unusual; nevertheless we need to be attentive in the diagnosis of the etiology of PA-AES.

2. Molecular mechanism of DENV and JEV co-infection

Co-infection with both viruses may occur in the single-cell types or different cells in the infected individuals. Simultaneous infection of target cells or different cell types by DENV and JEV defines the phenomenon of co-infection [18]. Both the viruses share common cell surface receptors expressed on target cell types such as DC-SIGN, mannose receptors, and CLEC5A [19]. On the other hand, virus can be internalized in the presence of non-neutralizing antibodies via Fcγ receptor-mediated endocytosis [20]. Clathrin-mediated endocytosis has been shown to be involved in the internalization of flaviviruses [21]. After internalization, the virus from the endocytic vesicles is delivered to the early endosomes [22]. Acidification of the endosomal

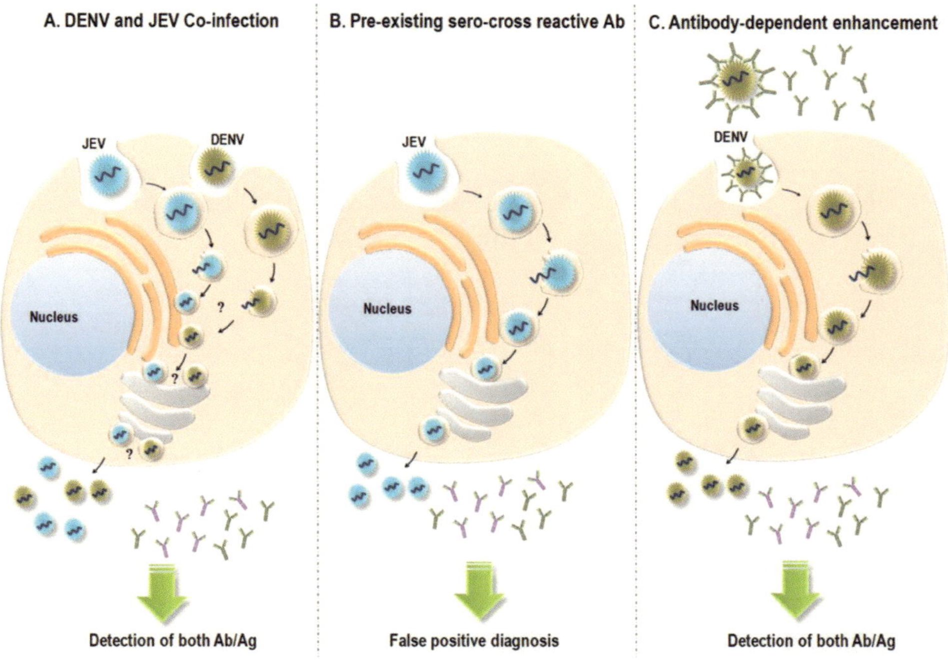

Figure 2.
DENV and JEV co-infection. The mechanism of co-infection has not been completely understood. Co-infection with DENV and JEV may occur in the single-cell types or different cells in the infected individuals. Co-infection results in the generation of antibodies against both viruses. However, detection of nucleic acids and antigens may confirm the phenomenon of co-infection (A). Upon infection, JEV is internalized by receptor-mediated endocytosis. The decrease in pH causes the fusion of viral and endosomal membrane which results in the release of viral RNA into the cytosol. The released viral genome is then translated prior to the commencement of replication. Virus maturation occurs at the Golgi complex and mature virus is released via the egress process. JEV infection in the hyperendemic area may result in false-positive diagnosis due to presence of pre-existing sero-cross-reactive antibody (B). Pre-existing sero-cross-reactive antibodies may bind to the viral particles upon infection which results in antibody-dependent enhancement of infection (C).

compartments causes trimerization of the envelope protein that results in the fusion of endosomes to the viral membrane and release of nucleocapsid in the cytosol [23].

The released viral genome is then translated prior to the commencement of replication [24]. The backbone of flaviviral genome is invariable which are of ~10 kb that codes for three structural capsid (C), premembrane (prM), and envelope (E) and seven nonstructural proteins NS1, NS2a, NS2b, NS3, NS4a, NS4b, and NS5. The viral genome encodes for 3400 amino acid long polyprotein which is arranged in the lumen endoplasmic reticulum where the replication takes place by the RNA-dependent RNA polymerase [25]. Replicated copies of the genome interact with viral proteins to form nucleocapsid. Immature virions enter into the secretary pathway where furin-mediated cleavage of prM results in the maturation of virus [26]. Mature virus is then released from the infected cells via the egress process [27]. The conventional mechanism of pathogenesis and viral replication may not be followed in case of co-infection and may involve distinct process. In order to effectively control and treat the co-infection of DENV and JEV, we need to first understand the immunopathogenesis of dual infection in various cell and animal models. The probable phenomenon of DENV and JEV co-infection has been demonstrated in **Figure 2**.

3. Diagnostic schemes for dengue and Japanese encephalitis co-infection

JEV is the most documented causative agent of acute encephalitis syndrome (AES) [28]. DENV has also been considered among the top three etiological agents causing

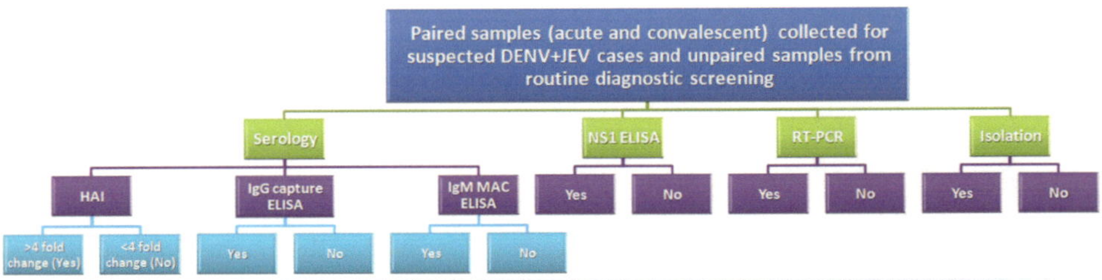

INTERPRETATION														
DENV					JEV					Co-infection (DENV + JEV)				
Virus Isolation	RT-PCR	NS1	Serology	Diagnosis	Virus Isolation	RT-PCR	NS1	Serology	Diagnosis	Virus Isolation	RT-PCR	NS1	Serology	Diagnosis
Y	?	?	?	Confirmed DENV	Y	?	?	?	Confirmed JEV	Y	?	?	?	Confirmed DENV+JEV
Y	Y	?	?	Confirmed DENV	Y	Y	?	?	Confirmed JEV	Y	Y	?	?	Confirmed DENV+JEV
Y	?	Y	?	Confirmed DENV	Y	?	Y	?	Confirmed JEV	Y	?	Y	?	Confirmed DENV+JEV
Y	?	?	Y	Confirmed DENV	Y	?	?	Y	Confirmed JEV	Y	?	?	Y	Confirmed DENV+JEV
?	Y	Y	?	Confirmed DENV	?	Y	Y	?	Confirmed JEV	?	Y	Y	?	Confirmed DENV+JEV
?	Y	?	Y	Confirmed DENV	?	Y	?	Y	Confirmed JEV	?	Y	?	Y	Confirmed DENV+JEV
?	?	Y	Y	Confirmed DENV	?	?	Y	Y	Confirmed JEV	?	?	Y	Y	Confirmed DENV+JEV
N	Y	N	N	Not DENV	N	Y	N	N	Not JEV	N	Y	N	N	Not DENV+JEV
N	N	Y	N	Not DENV	N	N	Y	N	Not JEV	N	N	Y	N	Not DENV+JEV
N	N	N	Y	Not DENV	N	N	N	Y	Not JEV	N	N	N	Y	Not DENV+JEV
N	N	N	N	Not DENV	N	N	N	N	Not JEV	N	N	N	N	Not DENV+JEV

Figure 3.
Laboratory diagnostic algorithms during DENV and JEV co-infection. Suspected cases of DENV and JEV co-infection can be decided by the above laboratory diagnostic algorithms of co-infection. Detection of IgG antibodies against both viruses may be considered as the previous exposure of the viruses, whereas detection of IgM or NS1 antigen suggests the recent or current infectious conditions. However, this should be further validated based on the nucleic acid-based tests such as RT-PCR and isolation of virus which may define the co-infectious condition in addition to the clinical correlation. "Y" indicates positive, "N" indicates negative, and "?" indicates inconclusive test report.

AES [29]. Broad spectrum of clinical features in the endemic areas of both viruses may dilute the encephalitis-like clinical presentation. Therefore, laboratory based diagnosis and discrimination of pathogenesis is crucial to understand. Detection of IgG antibodies against both viruses may be considered as the previous exposure of the viruses, whereas detection of IgM suggests the recent or current infectious conditions. However, this should be further validated based on the nucleic acid-based tests where detection of DENV and JEV nucleic acids defines the co-infectious condition.

Nucleic acid-based detection by RT-PCR for other probable arboviral infections such as Zika and Chikungunya can also be included which may overlap with the clinical manifestations of dengue or JE [30]. Although the clinical manifestations presented in the individual cases of DENV and JEV infections are distinct, the co-infection might be a complex situation to diagnose. Co-detection of serum antibodies against both viruses may not be the evidence of co-infection. Surveillance programs conducted in the hyperendemic areas of flaviviruses have reported at least 9% of co-infections cases [31]. Moreover, the MRI findings of DENV-infected patients may show the characteristic features of encephalitis as in case of JEV where the basal ganglia, thalamus, and midbrain are predominantly affected [32]. Considering the sero-cross-reactivity among flaviviruses, the dependence of serum-based diagnosis may give false-positive results. However, simultaneous detection of nucleic acid or viral-specific antigens in blood or CSF samples may define the incident of co-infection. The laboratory diagnostic algorithms during DENV and JEV co-infection have been depicted in **Figure 3**.

4. Treatments regimes for dengue and Japanese encephalitis co-infection

Viral infections have always been a global threat to mankind due to scarcity of effective antiviral drugs. Flaviviral infections are not the exception since there is no specific treatment available for both DENV and JEV [33]. The overall treatment relies on the symptomatic relief of the patients. Due to the complex and unclear pathogenesis of dual infection, the potential candidate drugs may not effective. Therefore, we need to look for the complementary and alternative medicine (CAM) in alliance with conventional medicines as the choice of treatment during co-infection.

In case of DENV infection, various forms of CAM have been used such as *Carica papaya* leaf extracts is the most accepted one. Platelet-activating factor receptor (PTAFR) gene has been shown to be upregulated upon consumption of *Carica papaya* leaf extracts or its juices [34]. In case of sever dengue infection, maintenance of body fluids volume of the patients is critical [35]. However, this may or may not be effective in case of co-infections. Recently, andrographolide has been shown to exhibit anti-DENV activity [36]. *Eupatorium perfoliatum* which is a homeopathic medicine has been shown to exhibit anti-DENV activity [37]. Luteolin has been shown to be effective during JEV infection which also exhibits direct virucidal activity [38]. Similarly, belladonna has been shown to be effective in chick embryos infected with JEV [39]. Several of the CAM-based therapies have been shown to be effective in case of JEV infection, but these have to be validated in case of co-infection.

5. Preventive strategies for dengue and Japanese encephalitis co-infection

To prevent the worldwide burden of DENV infection, the WHO has recently approved a tetravalent vaccine, Dengvaxia (CYD-TDV) in 20 countries. This has been designed by using the yellow fever vaccine backbone expressing the prM and envelope protein of DENV 1–4 serotypes [40]. In case of JEV, a live attenuated vaccine based on SA 14–14-2 has been used in China, India, Sri Lanka, Republic of Korea, and Thailand. Due to higher sero-cross-reactivity, the one vaccine may induce the other infection due to the antibody-dependent enhancement [41]. Therefore, to design an effective vaccine for co-infection, there is a need to understand the mechanism and probability of sero-cross-reactivity among the viruses. Apart from the vaccination, the personal preventive measures are always the paramount to prevent any vector-borne infections [42]. To prevent the mosquito biting, several protective measures include mosquito repellents, mosquito nets, and use of full sleeves cloths [43].

6. Conclusions

Genomic and proteomic sequence similarity among the flaviviruses causes the sero-cross-reactivity that leads to the phenomenon of antibody-dependent enhancement of infections. Incidence of DENV and JEV co-infection in the hyperendemic areas may be frequently reported. The diagnosis of co-infection should not rely on the presence of serum antibodies. However, simultaneous detection of nucleic acids or antigens may define the condition of co-infection. Clinical features may overlap in the patients infected with both viruses, and therefore we need to precisely distinguish the patients' clinical reports. Development of effective antivirals targeting both the viruses is the most imperative therapeutic strategy.

7. Future perspectives

Due to the similarity in the structural domains of the viral proteins, molecules may be designed to inhibit the action of viral proteins or enzymes. Similarly, vaccines may be designed to target the population living in the hyperendemic areas of flaviviruses. Peptide-based vaccines may be designed by using various immunoinformatics approaches by considering the consensus peptide sequences among the viruses. Apart from the vaccination, personal preventive measures are always recommended the best practice to reduce the chances of infections.

Acknowledgements

The authors are grateful to the Vice Chancellor, King George's Medical University (KGMU), Lucknow, India, for the encouragement and support for this work. SK Saxena is also supported by CCRH, Government of India, and US NIH grants: R37DA025576 and R01MH085259. The authors have no other relevant affiliations or financial involvement with any organization or entity with a financial interest in or financial conflict with the subject matter or materials discussed in the manuscript apart from those disclosed.

Author details

Shailendra K. Saxena*, Swatantra Kumar, Vimal K. Maurya and Madan L.B. Bhatt
Center for Advanced Research (CFAR)-Stem Cell/Cell Culture Unit, Faculty of Medicine, King George's Medical University, Lucknow, India

*Address all correspondence to: myedrsaxena@gmail.com

References

[1] Molyneux DH, Savioli L, Engels D. Neglected tropical diseases: Progress towards addressing the chronic pandemic. Lancet. 2017;**389**(10066):312-325

[2] Mitra AK, Mawson AR. Neglected tropical diseases: Epidemiology and global burden. Tropical Medicine and Infectious Disease. 2017;**2**(3):pii. E36

[3] Holbrook MR. Historical perspectives on Flavivirus research. Viruses. 2017;**9**(5):pii. E97

[4] Vogels CBF, Rückert C, Cavany SM, Perkins TA, Ebel GD, Grubaugh ND. Arbovirus coinfection and co-transmission: A neglected public health concern? PLoS Biology. 2019;**17**(1):e3000130

[5] Guo C, Zhou Z, Wen Z, Liu Y, Zeng C, Xiao D, et al. Global epidemiology of dengue outbreaks in 1990-2015: A systematic review and meta-analysis. Frontiers in Cellular and Infection Microbiology. 2017;7:317

[6] World Health Organization. Dengue and severe dengue. https://www.who.int/news-room/fact-sheets/detail/dengue-and-severe-dengue [Accessed: June 01, 2019]

[7] World Health Organization. Japanese encephalitis. https://www.who.int/news-room/fact-sheets/detail/japanese-encephalitis [Accessed: June 01, 2019]

[8] Daep CA, Muñoz-Jordán JL, Eugenin EA. Flaviviruses, an expanding threat in public health: Focus on dengue, west Nile, and Japanese encephalitis virus. Journal of Neurovirology. 2014;**20**(6):539-560

[9] Neufeldt CJ, Cortese M, Acosta EG, Bartenschlager R. Rewiring cellular networks by members of the Flaviviridae family. Nature Reviews. Microbiology. 2018;**16**(3):125-142

[10] Huang YJ, Higgs S, Horne KM, Vanlandingham DL. Flavivirus-mosquito interactions. Viruses. 2014;**6**(11):4703-4730

[11] Raj Y, Kumar S, Haikerwal A, Goel MM, Bhatt ML, Saxena SK. Current advances in Zika virus transmission: Urgency for effective therapeutics and prevention. American Journal of Infectious Diseases. 2017;**13**(2):13-20

[12] Saxena SK, Kumar S, Maurya VK. Pathogen-associated acute encephalitis syndrome: Therapeutics and management. Future Microbiology. 2019;**14**:259-262

[13] Saron WAA, Rathore APS, Ting L, Ooi EE, Low J, Abraham SN, et al. Flavivirus serocomplex cross-reactive immunity is protective by activating heterologous memory CD4 T cells. Science Advances. 2018;**4**(7):eaar4297

[14] Saito Y, Moi ML, Takeshita N, Lim CK, Shiba H, Hosono K, et al. Japanese encephalitis vaccine-facilitated dengue virus infection-enhancement antibody in adults. BMC Infectious Diseases. 2016;**16**(1):578

[15] Garg RK, Malhotra HS, Gupta A, Kumar N, Jain A. Concurrent dengue virus and Japanese encephalitis virus infection of the brain: Is it co-infection or co-detection? Infection. 2012;**40**(5):589-593

[16] Aggarwal A, Kumar P, Faridi MM. Neurological manifestation as presenting feature of dengue infection. Journal of Pediatric Neurosciences. 2015;**10**(1):76-77

[17] Tiroumourougane SV, Raghava P, Srinivasan S. Japanese viral encephalitis.

Postgraduate Medical Journal. 2002;**78**(918):205-215

[18] Salas-Benito JS, De Nova-Ocampo M. Viral interference and persistence in mosquito borne flaviviruses. Journal of Immunology Research. 2015;**2015**:873404

[19] Laureti M, Narayanan D, Rodriguez-Andres J, Fazakerley JK, Kedzierski L. Flavivirus receptors: Diversity, identity, and cell entry. Frontiers in Immunology. 2018;**9**:2180

[20] Slon Campos JL, Mongkolsapaya J, Screaton GR. The immune response against flaviviruses. Nature Immunology. 2018;**19**(11):1189-1198

[21] Piccini LE, Castilla V, Damonte EB. Dengue-3 virus entry into vero cells: Role of clathrin-mediated endocytosis in the outcome of infection. PLoS One. 2015;**10**(10):e0140824

[22] Hackett BA, Cherry S. Flavivirus internalization is regulated by a size-dependent endocytic pathway. Proceedings of the National Academy of Sciences of the United States of America. 2018;**115**(16):4246-4251

[23] Bressanelli S, Stiasny K, Allison SL, Stura EA, Duquerroy S, Lescar J, et al. Structure of a flavivirus envelope glycoprotein in its low-pH-induced membrane fusion conformation. The EMBO Journal. 2004;**23**(4):728-738

[24] Nour AM, Li Y, Wolenski J, Modis Y. Viral membrane fusion and nucleocapsid delivery into the cytoplasm are distinct events in some flaviviruses. PLoS Pathogens. 2013;**9**(9):e1003585

[25] Mazeaud C, Freppel W, Chatel-Chaix L. The multiples fates of the flavivirus RNA genome during pathogenesis. Frontiers in Genetics. 2018;**9**:595

[26] Plevka P, Battisti AJ, Junjhon J, Winkler DC, Holdaway HA, Keelapang P, et al. Maturation of flaviviruses starts from one or more icosahedrally independent nucleation centres. EMBO Reports. 2011;**12**(6):602-606

[27] Plevka P, Battisti AJ, Sheng J, Rossmann MG. Mechanism for maturation-related reorganization of flavivirus glycoproteins. Journal of Structural Biology. 2014;**185**(1):27-31

[28] Ghosh S, Basu A. Acute encephalitis syndrome in India: The changing scenario. Annals of Neurosciences. 2016;**23**(3):131-133

[29] Vasanthapuram R, Shahul Hameed SK, Desai A, Mani RS, Reddy V, Velayudhan A, et al. Dengue virus is an under-recognised causative agent of acute encephalitis syndrome (AES): Results from a four year AES surveillance study of Japanese encephalitis in selected states of India. International Journal Infectious Diseases. 2019;**84S**(2019):S19-S24

[30] Paixão ES, Teixeira MG, Rodrigues LC. Zika, chikungunya and dengue: The causes and threats of new and re-emerging arboviral diseases. BMJ Global Health. 2018;**3**(Suppl 1):e000530

[31] Singh KP, Mishra G, Jain P, Pandey N, Nagar R, Gupta S, et al. Co-positivity of anti-dengue virus and anti-Japanese encephalitis virus IgM in endemic area: co-infection or cross reactivity? Asian Pacific Journal of Tropical Medicine. 2014;7(2):124-129

[32] Verma R. MRI features of Japanese encephalitis. BML Case Reports. 2012; 2012. pii: bcr0320126088

[33] Wang S, Liu Y, Guo J, Wang P, Zhang L, Xiao G, Wang W. Screening of FDA-approved drugs for inhibitors of Japanese encephalitis virus infection.

Journal of Virology. 2017;**91**(21):pii. e01055-17

[34] Sarala N, Paknikar S. Papaya extract to treat dengue: A novel therapeutic option? Annals of Medical and Health Sciences Research. 2014;**4**(3):320-324

[35] Hung NT. Fluid management for dengue in children. Paediatrics and International Child Health. 2012;**32**(Suppl 1):39-42

[36] Panraksa P, Ramphan S, Khongwichit S, Smith DR. Activity of andrographolide against dengue virus. Antiviral Research. 2017;**139**:69-78

[37] Saxena SK, Haikerwal A, Gadugu S, Bhatt ML. Complementary and alternative medicine in alliance with conventional medicine for dengue therapeutics and prevention. Future Virology. 2017;**12**(8):399-402

[38] Fan W, Qian S, Qian P, Li X. Antiviral activity of luteolin against Japanese encephalitis virus. Virus Research. 2016;**220**:112-116

[39] Chakraborty U, Katoch S, Sinha M, Nayak D, Khurana A, Manchanda RK, et al. Changes in viral load in different organs of Japanese encephalitis virus-infected chick embryo under the influence of belladonna 200C. Indian Journal of Research in Homoeopathy. 2018;**12**(2):75

[40] Clapham H, Wills B. Implementing a dengue vaccination programme-who, where and how? Transactions of the Royal Society of Tropical Medicine and Hygiene. 2018;**112**(8):367-368

[41] Ginsburg AS, Meghani A, Halstead SB, Yaich M. Use of the live attenuated Japanese encephalitis vaccine SA 14-14-2 in children: A review of safety and tolerability studies. Human Vaccines & Immunotherapeutics. 2017;**13**(10):2222-2231

[42] Demers J, Bewick S, Calabrese J, Fagan WF. Dynamic modelling of personal protection control strategies for vector-borne disease limits the role of diversity amplification. Journal of the Royal Society Interface. 2018;**15**(145):pii. 20180166

[43] Tangena JA, Thammavong P, Chonephetsarath S, Logan JG, Brey PT, Lindsay SW. Field evaluation of personal protection methods against outdoor-biting mosquitoes in Lao PDR. Parasites & Vectors. 2018;**11**(1):661

Chapter 3

Diagnosis and Molecular Characterization of Chikungunya Virus Infections

Marta E. Álvarez-Argüelles, Susana Rojo Alba, Mercedes Rodríguez Pérez, Jose Antonio Boga Riveiro and Santiago Melón García

Abstract

In recent years, large-scale outbreaks of chikungunya arbovirus (CHIKV), which is transmitted by the *Aedes* mosquito, have enabled the rapid propagation of the virus across the world. After acute infection phase with commonly fever, joint pain, headache, or rash, chronic rheumatism (arthralgia or myalgia, anorexia, and concentration disorders) up to 40% of cases is observed. The chronic form is defined by symptoms persisting for more than 3 months, and up to years, after initial diagnosis. Chronic discomfort has been linked to one of the four genotypes described. These genotypes represent different geographic lineages (classification based on partial sequence of viral E1 glycoprotein): West African, East-Central-South-African (ECSA), ECSA-diverged or Indian Ocean Lineage (IOL), and Asian. The first marker detected in CHIK infection is the viral RNA, usually by reverse transcription-polymerase chain reaction (RT-PCR). This marker can be identified in samples within 8 days of symptom onset. The infection can also be diagnosed with serological testing to detect CHIKV-specific immunoglobulin IgG and/or IgM. Sequencing studies can determine the infecting genotype.

Keywords: chikungunya, genotype, chronic

1. Introduction

Chikungunya virus (CHIKV) is an emerging mosquito-borne alphavirus that causes severe acute febrile infection, often debilitating polyarthralgias and arthritis [1], and its symptoms are similar. The name chikungunya is derived from an African language *makonde* which means "that which bends up" or "stooped walk" because of the incapacitating arthralgia caused by the disease.

Chikungunya virus, the first reported case of which was in Tanzania in 1952 [2], is endemic in certain parts of West Africa, human serosurveys having identified antibodies to chikungunya virus in 35–50% of the population in some areas [3, 4].

1.1 Epidemiology, structure, and classification of chikungunya

Since 2004 CHIKV has spread into novel locations, with outbreaks having occurred in other parts of Africa as well as Asia, Europe, and the islands of the Indian and Pacific Oceans, and more recently in the Americas, mostly during the tropical rainy season. The risk of CHIKV being imported into further new areas is ever present because of the high attack rates, which affect between one-third to three-quarters of the population in areas where the virus is circulating, associated with the recurrence of epidemics, along with the high levels of viremia in infected humans and the worldwide distribution of the vectors, *Aedes aegypti* and *Aedes albopictus* [4]. Infected travelers can import chikungunya into new areas [1, 5–7], and in areas with *A. aegypti* and/or *A. albopictus* mosquitoes, local transmission can follow.

CHIKV multiple outbreaks have been identified as a cause of dengue-like illness with arthralgia in Africa and febrile hemorrhagic disease in Asia [2]. Although outbreaks of CHIKV were limited from the 1970s onward, in 2004–2005 the virus was detected in Kenya and the islands of the Indian Ocean in 2004–2005 [4, 8–10], and in the last decade, there have been massive outbreaks in new areas as well as in those where the virus is endemic [11]. What is more, local transmission of CHIKV has also been reported for the first time in parts of Europe, Asia [12], Australia [13], and America [9, 14, 15].

In the Americas, autochthonous CHIKV transmission was first reported in the Caribbean, on the island of St. Martin, in December 2013 [16], from which it is known to have spread to 45 countries or regions in Central/South/North America, where, according to the Pan American Health Organization, there had been 2 million suspected cases by 2014 [17]. It was detected in Central and South America in 2014, where there have since been multiple widescale outbreaks [13, 17], and between June and November of that same year, cases were reported in people returning to Northwest Italy from the Caribbean and Central America, even though there had been no reported cases of CHIKF in either region for 3 years [18]. More recently, in 2016–2017, autochthonous CHIKV transmission was reported in India [19], Pakistan [20], and Italy [21]. It can be assumed that the combination of increased global travel and trade, the wide distribution of the mosquito vectors, and a lack of herd immunity have all contributed to the introduction and rapid spread of CHIKV in naïve populations.

Dengue and *Zika* viruses are transmitted by the same mosquito vectors as chikungunya so all three viruses can co-circulate in a geographic region, and coinfections have been documented [22, 23]. This clearly has implications for diagnosis in the laboratory.

CHIKV belongs to the *Togaviridae* family, genus *Alphavirus*, within the Semliki Forest antigenic complex. Among the other members of this antigenic complex are the Mayaro, O'Nyong-nyong, and Ross River viruses, all of which are capable of causing disease in humans [24].

Chikungunya is a positive-sense single-stranded RNA virus with approximately 12 kb. It is spherical in shape and has a diameter of about 70 nm. The viral particle comprises 240 copies of the capsid protein contained within a lipid bilayer envelope which has 80 trimer-shaped spikes formed by E1 and E2 glycoproteins protruding from it [25]. There are two open reading frames (ORFs) in the genome: the 5'ORF (genomic RNA) is responsible for encoding the nonstructural proteins nsP1, nsP2, nsP3, and nsP4, and the 3'ORF (subgenomic RNA) is responsible for encoding a polyprotein that is processed into the structural capsid and envelope proteins (E1 and E2) and two peptides (E3 and 6 K) [26].

Several CHIKV genotypes which have been described are shown below: East-Central-South-African (ECSA) isolates which comprise the East, Central and South African, and West Africa isolates (West Africa) and Asian isolates (Asian). The Indian Ocean Lineage (IOL) was identified in 2004 as a descendant of the ECSA lineage [27, 28].

1.1.1 Chikungunya genotypes

CHIKV can be genetically classified into three major lineages: West African (WA); East, Central, and South African (ECSA); and Asian. Prior to 2004, these were rarely found outside the geographic limits implied by their names. The epidemics subsequent to 2004 were mainly due to isolates forming a distinct clade within the ECSA lineage [29], likely originating in eastern Kenya before spreading to cause large outbreaks affecting millions in islands of the Indian Ocean, India, and Asia [30], as well as numerous imported cases in previously nonendemic regions, including Europe and the Americas. More recently, since 2013, the Asian genotype has also caused significant outbreaks in the Caribbean and the Americas.

Additionally, the Indian Ocean (IOL) sublineage emerged within the ECSA clade, and the Asian/American sublineage emerged within the Asian clade [31, 32].

While differences in epidemiological and pathological characteristics among outbreaks involving different CHIKV lineages and sublineages have been suggested, few targeted investigations comparing lineage virulence levels have been reported.

The most important clades in terms of public health impact are the Asian lineage (including Asian/American) and the IOL sublineage, as well as some other ECSA lineage strains responsible for African outbreaks. They are responsible for multiple CHIKV outbreaks over the last 15 years involving millions of people [29, 32, 33], which continue to arise in Asia and Africa [34, 35].

CHIKV phylogenetic analysis, based on previous work speculating on the existence of distinct lineages [36], has established that the three principal currently circulating genotypes emerged from a common ancestor less than 500 years ago and that the ECSA and Asian genotypes separated within the past 150 years [29].

West African genotype is particularly well adapted to sylvatic mosquitoes or to a certain vector-host combination within the sylvatic cycle.

The Asian genotype that once circulated in India during the 1950s and 1960s formed a clade that was phylogenetically distinct from the Southeast Asian (SEA) strains that continue to circulate today. There is a remarkable spatial and temporal pattern in the evolution of the SEA lineage, spreading from Thailand to Indonesia and then to the Philippines and the South Pacific.

2. Transmission, pathogenesis, clinical disease, and differential diagnosis

Chikungunya virus is transmitted to people, as mentioned above, primarily via mosquito bites (primarily during the day but also at night). Mosquitoes become infected when they feed on a person already infected with the virus and then spread the virus to other people via biting, after the virus reaches the mosquito salivary glands. Other less-frequent routes of transmission are through blood products, organ transplantation, and maternal-fetal.

Pregnant women infected with CHIKV are not at increased risk of atypical or severe disease, but maternal CHIKV infection has been associated with miscarriage in the first trimester [16, 37, 38]. However, when maternal infection occurs toward the end of pregnancy, only 12% of newborns are expected to be symptomatic, clinical manifestations—fever, poor feeding, tenderness, unexplained apnea, peripheral edema, thrombocytopenia, and rash—appearing 3–7 days after delivery [37, 39]. More severe symptoms have also been observed, such as encephalopathy and myocardial disease, and neurocognitive development was found to be poor in children with perinatal CHIKV infection [40].

2.1 Clinical disease

The "natural" history of symptomatic CHIKV infection has been classified into three phases: acute, post-acute, and chronic.

Acute phase is considered the first 3 weeks of clinical manifestations. The incubation period is 3–7 days (range 1–14 days), and clinical manifestations begin abruptly, usually with high fever (>39°C), during 3–5 days (range 1–10 days), and malaise [41]. More than 85% of patients are symptomatic [1]. The duration of acute phase is usually 7–10 days.

Polyarthralgia, commonly bilateral and symmetric, begins 2–5 days after onset of fever and involves multiple joints: hands (50–76% of infected individuals), wrists (29–81%), ankles (41–68%), and axial skeleton (34–52%) [42, 43]. Pain may be intense and disabling, leading to immobilization.

Rash (maculopapular) has been reported in 40–75% of patients [43] and pruritus in 25–50% of patients.

Serious complications are not common, except in patients older than 65 years and patients with underlying pathologies, where the infection and symptoms can contribute to the cause of death. These severe forms usually involve the central nervous system, respiratory system, and urinary system.

Most patients recover fully, but in some cases joint pain may persist, or the patient experiences relapses of signs and symptoms for several months or even years [26].

In the *post-acute phase*, only a small proportion of patients remain completely asymptomatic 2–3 weeks after the onset of disease [44]. Generally, most patients exhibit only transitory improvements in their clinical condition, and relapses occur after a brief "healing" period. Most studies have indicated that, on average, clinical manifestations persist in 50–90% of patients after the second or third week, and the percentage of patients with persistent polyarthralgia after the acute phase of CHIKV infection is more frequent in those older than 40 years and in women [45].

Clinical manifestations observed during the post-acute phase, which indicate the persistence of the initial inflammatory process, include arthritis/arthralgia, edematous polyarthritis of fingers and toes, morning pain and stiffness, and severe tenosynovitis [42].

A set of nonspecific clinical manifestations that are not always associated with CHIKV usually occurs, such as chronic fatigue, changes in skin color, alopecia, decompensated endocrine and metabolic diseases, as well as the decompensation of other preexisting chronic diseases, depression, and anxiety [44].

Chronic phase: It is estimated that the percentage of patients infected with chikungunya virus who progress to chronic phase (more than 3 months) varies from 40 to 80% [45–47], and they may endure clinical manifestations for a few months or even years [44]. Although no clear evidence exists to explain the pathogenesis of persistent symptoms following infection, two hypotheses have been proposed: (a) That viral and/or antigenic debris remains in the tissues of joints and muscles. Unfortunately, to date, the virus has not been isolated from such tissue. However, CHIKV proteins have been found in macrophages and muscle cell tissue of relapsing CHIKV patients, supporting the notion that there may be low-grade replication of the virus or non-replicative viral debris present. (b) That infection triggers a persistent immune response. Studies are underway with mouse models to determine whether, and in what way, immunological mechanisms might be altered in patients with persistent symptoms [48, 49].

Chronic phase sufferers can be divided into three groups in terms of disease progression: those whose symptoms disappear either spontaneously or following treatment and who have no long-term complications, which accounts for the majority of such cases; a group who experiences prolonged and persistence generalized clinical symptoms, with or without joint problems; and another set of patients in whom the degenerative or inflammatory process is exacerbated and their condition becomes serious [44].

Twenty-five percent of CHIKV cases have been estimated to result in chronic inflammatory rheumatism, although this study did not address the issue of differences between genotypes [50]. Other symptoms, such as chronic pain, mental health issues, and nonspecific manifestations, are also common in this phase [51–54], with arthralgia and arthritis with pain accompanied by articular edema or morning joint stiffness being the most frequent clinical manifestations [55]. Tenosynovitis is also frequent (with two or more tendons affected), and less common symptoms are fatigue and neuritis [44]. Clearly the daily life of patients with long-term chronic CHIKV symptoms is considerably impacted [54], and interestingly there is some evidence that the incidence of chronic symptoms is greater in high-income than low-income countries, albeit that the confidence intervals overlapped [54]. These same authors did consider the relationship between virus genotype and self-reported chronic discomfort and found this symptom to be less prevalent in those infected by the ECSA group, followed by those carrying the Asian strain. The highest prevalence was linked to the ECSA-diverged/IOL genotypes, though there was overlap with the Asian strain.

There is no commercial vaccine against CHIKV, although development is underway [56–58] and there is no specific antiviral therapy for acute infection. Treatment in this phase consists of supportive care for as long as the infection is confirmed. It is, however, known that systemic glucocorticoids and other immunosuppressive medications should be avoided in patients during acute infection [44].

The management of persistent or relapse symptoms, particularly joint disease, depends upon the duration of the symptoms. Treatment with anti-inflammatory drugs and analgesics is appropriate in the acute phase. On the other hand, for symptoms persisting for more than 3 months after infection, the use of disease-modifying antirheumatic drug (DMARD) therapy, such as methotrexate (MTX) and hydroxychloroquine [44], or, as an alternative, physiotherapy is indicated [59].

2.2 Differential diagnosis

Fever and polyarthralgia are key symptoms of CHIKV infection but are far from being reliable diagnostic markers since they have a sensitivity of only 84%, a positive predictive value (PPV) of 71%, and an 83% negative predictive value (NPV) [25]. Thus differential diagnosis of both the acute and the chronic manifestations of the disease can be complex and take time due to the nonspecific nature of the typical symptoms of arthralgia, high fever, and rash. The shared vectors, as well as symptoms, of CHIKV and the DENV, ZK, O'nyong-nyong, and Mayaro viruses, as well as the fact that the viruses all co-exist and are known to co-infect, mean that they must all be ruled out in the differential diagnosis.

Therefore, it is difficult to differentiate from those of other febrile illnesses or be misdiagnosed in areas where dengue occurs. Other infections that should be considered include malaria, yellow fever, leptospirosis, measles, mononucleosis, or African tick bite fever.

An additional diagnostic complication is the similarity of chronic arthralgia caused by chikungunya fever with other more common causes, and it has been demonstrated that patients with underlying joint disease prior to CHIKV infection have worse prognosis and increased morbidity [60]. Differential serological diagnosis includes the exclusion of rheumatoid and systemic arthritis, lupus erythematosus Reiter arthritis, rheumatoid arthritis, and hepatitis C.

It is thus clear that differential diagnosis is essential to establish CHIKV infection and ensure the appropriate public health response as well as the optimal treatment regime for the patient. Employing a single PCR which targets all three infectious agents (CHIKV, DENV, ZV), available from US Centers for Disease Control and Prevention (CDC) and approved laboratories, would expediate diagnosis [61–64].

3. Diagnosis

Chikungunya virus infection should be suspected in patients with acute onset of fever and polyarthralgia and who meet the relevant epidemiologic exposure criteria (residence in or travel to an area where mosquito-borne transmission of chikungunya virus infection has been reported).

The laboratory diagnosis of CHIKV infection can be achieved in the majority of cases by following two different strategies: the detection of viral RNA (virological diagnosis) and the identification of the specific immune response (serological diagnosis). To this end, choosing the appropriate timing of specimen collection and of the use of the most suitable diagnostic methodologies is crucial for accurate diagnosis. The algorithm developed by the US Center for Disease Control and Prevention (CDC) to diagnose CHIKV infections is based on the characteristics of CHIKV infection and the timing of specimen collection (**Figure 1**).

CHIKV replicates rapidly to high titers in the host, and viral RNA generally can be detected by real-time RT-PCR in the first week after onset of clinical illness, while immunoglobulin M (IgM) antibodies are normally detectable in serum by days 5–7 after onset of illness [65]. Consequently, the kinetic replication and pathogenesis of CHIKV infection, including the duration of viremia and the response of the host immune response, should be considered when selecting the appropriate diagnostic tests [66]. Molecular assays (TaqMan real-time PCR, RT-LAMP assay, and reverse transcription PCR) are more sensitive in the early stage of chikungunya fever (2–5 days p.o.i.) when CHIKV-specific IgM is not yet detectable. In the later stages of chikungunya fever (>5 days p.o.i.), CHIKV-specific IgM is a more reliable indicator.

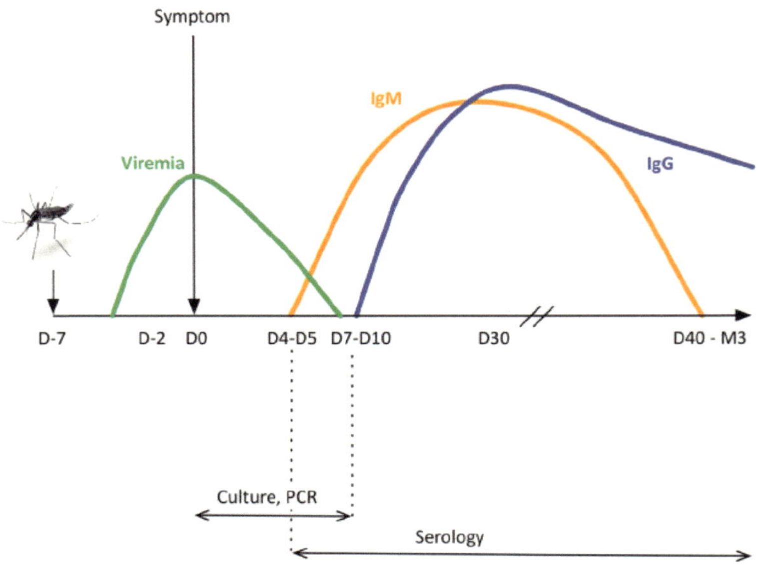

Figure 1.
Time course of chikungunya virus viremia and immune response. Source of CDC.

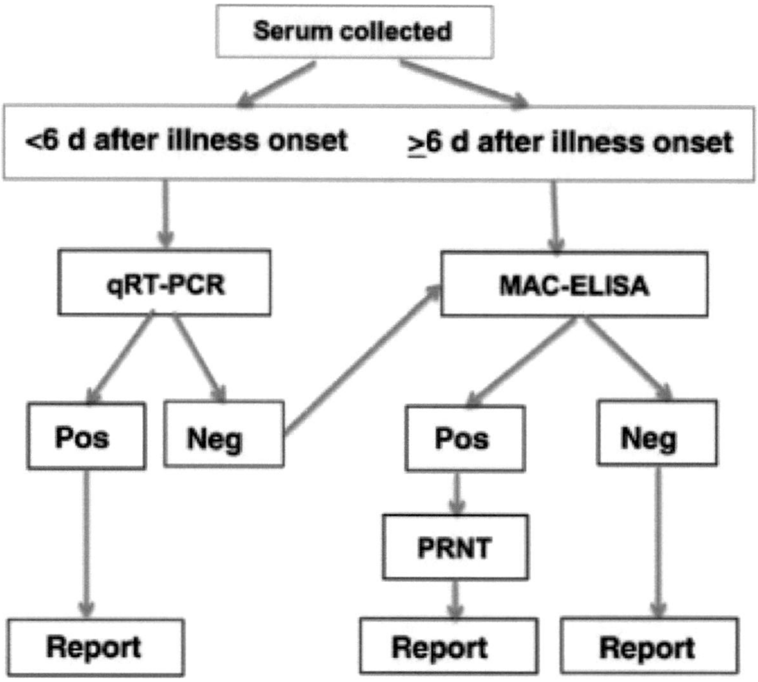

Figure 2.
The Centers for Disease Control and Prevention diagnostic testing algorithm for detection of chikungunya virus infection. Source of CDC.

In the CHIKV testing algorithm developed by the CDC arbovirus diagnostic laboratory, samples collected <6 days after onset of illness are first tested by virological methods (CHIKV real-time RT-PCR using two different set primers/probe that were developed to detect different genotypes (**Figure 2**)).

The CDC guidelines indicate that samples collected on or after day 6 of illness and samples with negative real-time RT-PCR results are tested by serological methods (the CHIKV IgM antibody-capture enzyme-linked immunosorbent assay (MAC-ELISA) or an indirect fluorescent antibody assay (IFA) and plaque reduction hemagglutination test as confirmation) [67–70].

3.1 Types of samples for chikungunya infection diagnosis

Samples for chikungunya diagnosis have to be collected as soon as possible. Two different types of sample are suitable for virological and/or serological diagnosis.

Viral diagnosis depends on the characteristics of CHIKV infection and the time elapsed since the viral infection, the type of patient (e.g., fetus, pregnant, etc.), and clinical manifestation of infection. Virological diagnosis can be made using samples of blood (whole blood, plasma, or serum), urine, blister fluid, cerebrospinal fluid, amniotic fluid, or tissues such as the placenta and brain, among others.

Samples must be collected in strictly aseptic conditions and in the right container: sterile recipients for fluids and with transport viral medium for the others (blisters, biopsies, swabs, etc.).

Samples need to be sent to the laboratory quickly.

The best type of tube for serological diagnosis is serum separator. Heparin and EDTA are unsuitable for antibodies CHIK testing [71]. Serum used for serological test can be used for virological diagnosis, but plasma or whole blood (leukocytes) is preferable.

3.2 Virological diagnosis

As was described above, for virological diagnosis it is important to know the pathogenesis and the infection kinetics. The RNA viruses are found in plasma or serum specimens between 2 and 6 days following onset of fever, which corresponds to the period of incubation [41]. Viral load can subsequently rapidly reach up to $10^8/10^9$ genome copies/ml of blood [1, 26, 37].

Complete virions as well as viral fragments (antigen or genome) are frequent in this phase, although replication later declines. In line with this kinetic replication, three methods can be used in the laboratory: viral isolation and antigen or genomic detection.

3.2.1 Viral isolation

Viral isolation is generally a research tool [71–73]. For viral culture it is essential to preserve the complete virion. Culture sensitivity for chikungunya virus is high only in early infection (during the viremic phase) but drops 5 days after onset of illness. As a result, virus isolation is rarely used in the diagnosis of CHIKV infection because low sensitivity occurs after only a few days post-infection, and it is time-consuming and laborious procedure. However, it does allow for the identification of the viral strain and can be important for epidemiologic and research purposes. Samples where chikungunya virus is suspected should be handled under Biosafety Level (BSL) 3 conditions.

A wide variety of cells are used for in vitro CHIKV cultures in order to assess the full scope of the disease, including primary human skeletal muscle myoblasts [74], human blood monocytes [75], African green monkey kidney (Vero-E6) cells [76], and C6/36 (*Aedes albopictus* clone cells). Of particular interest, given the known tropism of chronic CHIKV for bone and synovial tissues, is the use of primary human fibroblast-like synoviocytes [77] and human osteoblasts.

Culture on HEL cells is more sensitive, and the presence of a cytopathic effect can be observed earlier than in Vero cells [78].

These cultures all need to be maintained under standard conditions.

3.2.2 Antigen detection

There are commercial immunochromatography antigen detection kits which detect CHIKV with high sensitivity in the early phase (up to 4–5 days after the onset of fever, when blood-enveloping proteins are still present). These tests also have high specificity since no cross-reactions with dengue virus are known to exist, and the method is straightforward and simple and does not require specially trained laboratory personnel [79].

However, a very important issue to consider is what genotype/s the tests are capable of detecting since not all detect all the known genotypes. Thus the geographical area from which the patient comes, meaning they are more likely to have one genotype or another, needs to be taken into account for accurate diagnosis (e.g., Okabayashi's immunochromatography only detects the Asian genotype) [80].

These methods are therefore, generally, sensitivity compromised.

3.2.3 Genomic detection (RT-PCR)

The diagnosis of CHIKV infection in the acute phase of infection is typically performed by the detection of viral RNA in plasma or serum (or other sample types) by RT-PCR. The viral RNA can be detected by various molecular methods, such as nested and real-time PCRs [37].

Conventional and real-time PCRs have been used to amplify nsP1, nsP2, or even envelope protein genes (E3, E2, or E1) [81, 82].

Molecular diagnostic tests used for the detection of CHIKV include reverse transcription (RT) and amplification (PCR) assay of fragments in the nsP1, nsP2, nsP3, nsP4, or E1 regions of the CHIKV genome, in general by real-time [65, 82–86]. Labeled probes or SYBR Green is used for real-time quantification of the amplified PCR products [87, 88]. In these assays, the limits of detection range between 0.5 and 1.5 log10 RNA copies/reaction. Although the detection of positive-strand RNA is commonly used for diagnostic purposes, assays to detect negative-strand CHIKV RNA have also been developed. These include strand-specific quantitative RT-PCRs for nsP1 [89] and nsP3 [90], which use a tagged-primer system to improve PCR specificity and accuracy. In comparison to the detection of positive-strand RNA, the detection limit for negative-strand RNA assays is slightly decreased, 3 log10 RNA copies [91].

While there is an ever-present possibility of CHIKV spreading further in developed countries in the Americas and Europe, CHIKV still predominantly occurs in resource-limited countries. *Loop-mediated isothermal amplification* (LAMP) amplifies nucleic acid under isothermal conditions without the use of a thermal cycler and is a fast, specific, and cost-effective technique [92]; LAMP represents a cheaper alternative amplification method, albeit with lower sensitivity than real-time RT-PCR. Monitoring by turbidity as well as observation of color change after adding SYBR Green has also been described for the detection of CHIKV [85, 92]. Visualization is made with the naked eye, meaning no sophisticated equipment is required, and thus LAMP is especially useful in developing countries or in field studies.

Another method, *microfluidic lab-on-chip* integrating multiplex molecular amplification and DNA microarray hybridization, has been developed for the simultaneous detection of 26 globally important tropical pathogens such as CHIKV, *Dengue virus* (DENV), and other arboviruses [93]. Such diagnostic capacity provides an effective and rapid means to establish the presence of specific potential pathogens.

The CDC protocol for chikungunya infection diagnosis uses two RT-PCRs. The nucleotide sequences of the two sets of primers and probes used are listed in **Table 1** [94, 95]. The 3855 primer/probe set is specific to the ECSA genotypes although it is

Primer/genome 5′ position	Nucleotide sequence
CHIKV3855F	GAGCATACGGTTACGCAGATAG
CHIKV3957C	TACTGGTGATACATGGTGGTTTC + TGCTGGTGACACATGGTGGTTTC
CHIKV3886FAM (probe)	ACGAGTAATCTGCGTACTGGGACGTA + ACGAGTCATCTGCGTATTGGGACGCA
CHIK856F	ACCATCGGTGTTCCATCTAAAG
CHIK962C	GCCTGGGCTCATCGTTATT
CHIK908FAM (probe)	ACAGTGGTTTCGTGTGAGGGCTAC

Table 1.
Chikungunya virus oligonucleotide primers and probes used in the Centers for Disease Control and Prevention real-time reverse transcription-polymerase chain reaction assays designed to detect CHIKV Asian genotype strains.

Virus	Name	Sequence (5′-3′)	Amplicon size
	DEN.ZIK-TR-S	AAGGACTAGAGGTTAGAGGAGACCC	
Dengue	DEN-TR-A	GAGACAGCAGGATCTCTGGTCT	83 bp
	DEN-FAM	AACAGCATATTGACGCTGG	
	DEN.ZIK-TR-S	AAGGACTAGAGGTTAGAGGAGACCC	
Zika	ZIK-TR-A3	GGCCAGCGTGGTGGAA	96 bp
	ZIK-FAM	AAACAGCATATTGACG	
	CHK-TR-S	CGGCGACCATTTGTGATCA	
Chikungunya	CHK-TR-A	TTCGTATTCCGTTGCGTTCTG	127 bp
	CHK-FAM	CCGGCATCCTTGCTA	
	WN.FA-TR-S	GGCTGGGGCAAYGGCT	
Yellow fever	FA-TR-A	CCTCAAACAAACTCATGGATTTG	91 bp
	WN-FA-FAM	CATGCGCCAAATT	
	WN.FA-TR-S	GGCTGGGGCAAYGGCT	
West Nile	WN-TR-A	CAAGATGGTTCTTCCTATTGCCT	96 bp
	WN-FA-FAM	CATGCGCCAAATT	

Table 2.
Primers and probes used to detect DENV, CHIKV, ZIKV, YFV, and WNV.

capable of detecting both Asian and ECSA genotypes [95]. The 856 primer/probe set targets the Asian genotype, which has a slightly higher sensitivity than the 3855 set, which is prevalent in the Caribbean. This elevated sensitivity makes it a valuable tool for confirming diagnosis in samples where CHIKV RNA levels are reduced. These characteristics should be taken into account for testing protocols (i.e., which sets to use and in what order).

In our experience "in-house" real-time PCR is a useful tool in the chikungunya diagnosis. As such, proprietary primers and probe have been designed (**Table 2**) for CHIKV. In addition, for the syndromic diagnosis of imported viral diseases, our in-house RT-PCR can also detect other arboviruses such as Zika, dengue, yellow fever, and West Nile (**Table 2**) with sensitivities/specificities comparable to, or even superior to, commercially available techniques [63].

Genomic analysis is also used to classify and characterize viruses usually by Sanger sequencing method.

The sequencing of envelope E1 (viral structural glycoprotein) is often used for phylogenetic analysis. The three principal strains of CHIKV (ECSA, West African, and Asian) have been typed by nucleotide sequencing of a portion of the E1 region using RT-PCR [96].

Using sequencing studies to examine genomic evolution, it has been determined that global chikungunya outbreaks since 2005 have occurred as a result of a mutation of the ECSA lineage: an alanine-to-valine substitution in the E1 envelope glycoprotein at position 226 (A226V), which enabled the virus to acquire a new mosquito vector, *A. albopictus,* commonly known as the Asian tiger mosquito, conferring increased virus adaptation and replication ability in *Aedes albopictus*.

There are also specific regions that showed nucleotide variability and novel mutations making them suitable for phylogenetic analysis in nsP2 and E2 CHIKV regions [97].

3.3 Serological diagnosis

A variety of serological methods (hemagglutination inhibition, ELISA, complement fixation, and neutralization of viral infectivity using reference serum samples) can be used to characterize the alphavirus species [15, 98]. A fourfold increase in levels of CHIK virus IgG antibody in serum samples taken during the acute and the recovery phase is required to serodiagnosis. However, it is often problematic to collect paired samples, and so the existence of CHIKV-specific IgM antibodies in acute-phase samples is used instead. Also, patient serum coupled with neutralization by reference serum can be taken as definitive proof of the presence of CHIKV.

Several serological assays have been developed, the large majority of which demonstrate high reliability and specificity. The most common first-line serological techniques used for CHIKV diagnosis are the enzyme-linked immunosorbent assay (ELISA) and indirect immunofluorescence (IFA) assays, and the most suitable sample type is serum, generally using 1/100 dilutions. Commercially available ELISA tests, for example, have been shown to demonstrate high sensitivity (ranging from 82 to 88%) and specificity in samples from recovering patients [99, 100].

The presence of IgM antibodies indicates recent CHIKV infection [41], generally occurring in samples taken 2 weeks prior to patients becoming symptomatic. Detection of specific IgG antibodies, on the other hand, indicates previous CHIKV infection, which can be recent or as long ago as several months or years, given the persistence of anti-CHIKV IgG antibodies [1].

3.3.1 Enzyme-linked immunosorbent assay

CHIKV-specific IgM and IgG can be detected in serum using enzyme-linked immunosorbent assay immunocapture. The first antibodies detected in patients with chikungunya fever is CHIKV-specific IgM, which commonly appears 3–8 days after the onset of infection and may persist for several months to 2 years. After 4–10 days since onset of infection, the IgG antibodies become detectable in serum and may persist for years (**Figure 1**) [1] and be potentially lifelong. The chances of cross-reactivity between IgG and other viruses of the Semliki antigenic serocomplex are less now than in the past due to improvements in test design and procedure, but IgG seroconversion (greater than fourfold increase) is still recommended for reliable diagnosis. Furthermore, the existence of closely related alphaviruses in the area where the patient was infected necessitates the use of plaque reduction neutralization testing to confirm CHIKV infection [101].

ELISA is a rapid and sensitive method largely used for the detection of anti-CHIKV antibodies. The most common tests used for the diagnosis of CHIKV infection are IgM antibody-capture ELISA (MAC- ELISA) and indirect ELISA (i-ELISA) for the detection of type M (IgM) and type G (IgG) immunoglobulin, respectively [102]. A list of different commercially available ELISA tests is shown in **Table 3**.

Enzyme-linked immunosorbent assays can be used to confirm the presence of anti-CHIKV antibodies, with IgM antibody levels highest 3–5 weeks post-infection and persisting for up to 2 months.

ELISA is not, however, without its disadvantages: false-positives because of cross-reactivity with other alphaviruses (Ross River virus, Barmah Forest virus, and Sindbis virus [103]) and its sensitivity being much reduced (4–20%) in serum samples taken during the acute phase [104].

Company	IgM	IgG	Test
Euroimmun	+	+	ELISA
Novatec	+	/	IgM-capture ELISA
Novatec	/	+	ELISA
IBL	+	/	IgM-capture ELISA
IBL	/	+	IgG-capture ELISA
Abcam	+	+	ELISA
DRG	+	/	IgM-capture ELISA
DRG	/	+	ELISA
GenWay	+	/	IgM-capture ELISA
GenWay	/	+	ELISA
Standard diagnostic	+	+	ELISA
Euroimmun	+	+	IFA

Table 3.
Commercial diagnostic test available for serological diagnosis of CHIKV infection.

For these reasons, commercially available rapid diagnostic kits often do not provide as reliable results as RT-PCR because they all tend to detect host-derived anti-CHIKV IgM antibodies. Furthermore, since IgM antibodies are produced later in the course of infection than the antigen, this is a less sensitive test and as such can delay diagnosis and reduce the effectiveness of disease management [105].

3.3.2 Indirect immunofluorescence

IFA is an accurate and reliable technique widely used for the detection of specific anti-CHIK antibodies. IFA reveals the presence of type-specific antibodies against CHIKV by detecting the presence of virus antigens in infected cells.

The specificity of commercial IFA tests has been found to range from 75 to 100% in serum collected 5–6 days after infection [106]. That said IFA has some shortcomings in that it is laborious and the personnel carrying out the procedure need to be specially trained. In addition interpretation of the microscope examination results can be rather subjective, and there is no standardization between labs.

3.3.3 Antibody neutralization assay

The neutralization assay is generally used following ELISA or IFA results to confirm CHIKV. Neutralization involves the interaction of viral antigens and specific antibodies to block infection. The neutralization test requires the mixing of virus and serum, and the resulting mixture is then inoculated into cell culture. Inhibition of the virus can then be tested, using a variety of methods, after a number of days [107]. The microneutralization assay (MNA) evaluates the neutralizing antibodies. Although both methods have high specificity and sensitivity, there are disadvantages, namely, they are labor-intensive since only a small number of samples can be processed in each run and a Biosafety Level 3 laboratory (BSL-3) is required because live virus is being used.

The drawbacks to antibody testing include cross-reactivity with other alpha viruses and the problem of it not being able to distinguish between recent past and acute infection, as well as the fact that its sensitivity varies between clinical settings.

3.4 Diagnosis in other patients

Diagnosis is clearly always important for appropriate patient management, but it becomes crucial in several specific circumstances.

3.4.1 Transplantation or transfusion

CHIKV, like other arboviruses, can be transmitted by blood transfusion or through organ transplant from infected donors who were asymptomatic at the time of donation. Transmission via organ transplantation could also occur since chikungunya viremia (which may exceed 10^9 RNA copies/ml plasma) is likely prior to onset of symptoms [86, 108, 109].

In a case series of Rosso et al., 80% of the patients presented high viral load (>10^6 copies/ml), and none of the solid organ transplant patients with CHIKV infection developed graft rejection or died [110].

In these patients, blood and/or tissues are essential in the diagnosis.

3.4.2 Maternal-fetal transmission

Vertical transmission of CHIKV is a possibility and can affect the fetus, both congenital and perinatal infection having been demonstrated.

Congenital and perinatal CHIKV infections were reported following delivery to mothers with documented viremia accompanied by symptoms of CHIKF [16, 111, 112].

Vertical transmission rate of CHIKV has been estimated to range from 27.7 to 48.29%, and the same paper found transmission to be increased in mothers experiencing viremia at the time of birth. Neonatal symptoms were found to begin within 3–9 days postpartum, although there is no evidence of any link between birth method and incidence of congenital disease [113].

No link between CHIKV exposure in the first trimester of gestation and higher miscarriage risk or congenital malformation has been found to date [114, 115]. However, infection in the second or third trimester has been linked with increased fetal mortality, although the mechanism of this is unclear [111, 116]. Furthermore, a change in the evolution of neonates vertically infected with CHIKV has been seen following the spread of the virus to Indian Oceanic regions and Latin America in terms of the previously minor, self-limiting symptoms having been replaced by multiple severe manifestations and sometimes death [117].

Of particular note is the serious outbreak of CHIKV in 2006 in the Reunion Islands where complications were reported, including seizures and abnormal MRI scans [118, 119] as well as cardiac defects in almost 50% of patients [119]. In infants, these conditions can lead to death in the first year of life if swift and targeted medical intervention is not carried out [120, 121]. All patients in this outbreak who exhibited symptoms of neuroinvasive disease were infected with the A226V variant strain [122].

Virus infection in fetuses can be documented by positive RT-PCR in the amniotic fluid, and placenta, and in the cases of miscarriage, the involvement of CHIKV can be investigated in the brain or other fetal tissues [40].

3.4.3 Children

The first descriptions of CHIKF in children were made in the 1960s during outbreaks in India and South Asia [123–127]. In these younger patients, the infection presented as a febrile illness, with rash and joint pain or dengue-like illness, hemorrhagic fever, or CSF infection. Asian lineage infection of children resulted in a lower frequency of arthralgia than in those infected by the African lineages, although hemorrhagic fever was more frequent in children testing positive for the former [117].

Lately, in the regions surrounding the Indian Ocean and the expansion of CHIKV into the Western Hemisphere, CHIKV-WH infections in children and neonates are reported more frequently and with more severe syndromes and sequelae [117].

4. Summary

In recent years, large-scale outbreaks of the chikungunya arbovirus (CHIKV) have permitted rapid propagation of the virus across the globe. CHIKV is transmitted by the *Aedes* mosquito, and the acute infection phase typically results in fever, joint pain, headache or rash, and chronic rheumatism (arthralgia or myalgia, anorexia, and concentration disorders) in up to 40% of cases.

The chronic form is defined by symptoms which persist for more than 3 months, and up to years, after initial diagnosis. The negative impact of CHIKV infection on the patient's health-related quality of life is quite severe and is not limited to the acute disease, and the repercussions may last for several months after clinical recovery. The highest prevalence of chronic discomfort was linked to one of the four genotypes described. These genotypes represent different geographic lineages (classification based on partial sequence of viral E1 glycoprotein): West African, East-Central-South-African (ECSA), ECSA-diverged or Indian Ocean Lineage, and Asian lineage.

The first marker detected in CHIK infection is the viral RNA, usually by RT-PCR. This marker can be present in samples taken within 8 days of onset of the illness. After this initial acute phase, the infection can also be diagnosed by serological detection of CHIKV-IgG and/or IgM-specific immunoglobulin, and sequencing studies can determine the infecting genotype.

The correct diagnosis of chikungunya infection enables the disease progression to be better predicted and patients' treatment to be more effectively managed.

Author details

Marta E. Álvarez-Argüelles*, Susana Rojo Alba, Mercedes Rodríguez Pérez, Jose Antonio Boga Riveiro and Santiago Melón García
Microbiology Department, Hospital Universitario Central de Asturias, Oviedo, Spain

*Address all correspondence to: martaealvarez@gmail.com

References

[1] Weaver SC, Lecuit M. Chikungunya virus and the global spread of a mosquito-borne disease. New England Journal of Medicine. 2015;**372**:1231-1239

[2] Ross RW. The Newala epidemic: III. The virus: Isolation, pathogenic properties and relationship to the epidemic. Journal of Hygiene (London). 1956;**54**(2):177-191

[3] Chevillon C, Briant L, Renaud F, Devaux C. The chikungunya threat: An ecological and evolutionary perspective. Trends in Microbiology. 2008;**16**(2):80

[4] Staples JE, Breiman RF, Powers AM. Chikungunya fever: An epidemiological review of a re-emerging infectious disease. Clinical Infectious Diseases. 2009;**49**(6):942

[5] Charrel RN, de Lamballerie X, Raoult D. Chikungunya outbreaks—The globalization of vector-borne diseases. The New England Journal of Medicine. 2007;**356**:769

[6] Morens DM, Fauci AS. Chikungunya at the door--déjà vu all over again? The New England Journal of Medicine. 2014;**371**:885

[7] Rodriguez-Lucas C, Alvarez-Argüelles ME, Melon Garcia S, Boga Riveiro JA, Palacio Suarez A, Oña Navarro M. Development of a real time-PCR assay for chikungunya fever diagnosis. In: 26th European Congress of Clinical Microbiology and Infectious Diseases. Vol. 9-12. Amsterdam: Abril; 2016

[8] Mohan A, Kiran D, Manohar IC, Kumar DP. Epidemiology, clinical manifestations, and diagnosis of chikungunya fever: Lessons learned from the re-emerging epidemic. Indian Journal of Dermatology. 2010;**55**(1):54-53

[9] Gérardin P, Guernier V, Perrau J, Fianu A, Le Roux K, Grivard P, et al. Estimating chikungunya prevalence in La Réunion Island outbreak by serosurveys: Two methods for two critical times of the epidemic. BMC Infectious Diseases. 2008;**8**:99

[10] Chretien JP, Anyamba A, Bedno SA, Breiman RF, Sang R, Sergon K, et al. Drought-associated chikungunya emergence along coastal East Africa. The American Journal of Tropical Medicine and Hygiene. 2007;**76**(3):405-407

[11] Weaver SC, Forrester NL. Chikungunya: Evolutionary history and recent epidemic spread. Antiviral Research. 2015;**120**:32-39

[12] Wu D, Wu J, Zhang Q, Zhong H, Ke C, Deng X, et al. Chikungunya outbreak in Guangdong province, China. Emerging Infectious Diseases. 2010;**18**:493-495

[13] Van Bortel W, Dorleans F, Rosine J, Blateau A, Rousset D, Matheus S, et al. Chikungunya outbreak in the Caribbean region, December 2013 to March 2014, and the significance for Europe. Euro Surveillance. 2014;**19**(13): pii/20764

[14] Leparc-Goffart I, Nougairede A, Cassadou S, Prat C, de Lamballerie X. Chikungunya in the Americas. The Lancet. 2014;**383**(9916):514

[15] Morrison TE. Reemergence of chikungunya virus. Journal of Virology. 2014;**88**:11644-11647

[16] Lenglet Y, Barau G, Robillard PY, Randrianaivo H, Michault A, Bouveret A, et al. Chikungunya infection in pregnancy: Evidence for intrauterine infection in pregnant women and vertical transmission in the parturient. Survey of the Reunion Island outbreak. Journal de

Gynécologie Obstétrique et Biologie de la Reproduction (Paris). 2006;**35**:578

[17] PAN American Health Organization (PAHO). Chikungunya. World Health Organization (WHO); 2014. Available from: http://www.paho.org/hq/index.php?Itemid=40931 [Accessed: Nov 21, 2014]

[18] Burdino E, Ruggiero T, Milia MG, Proietti A, Sergi G, Torta I, et al. Travelers with chikungunya virus infection returning to Northwest Italy from the Caribbean and Central America during June–November 2014. Journal of Travel Medicine. 2015;**22**(5):341-344

[19] Kaur N, Jain J, Kumar A, Narang M, Zakaria MK, Marcello A, et al. Chikungunya outbreak in Delhi, India, 2016: Report on coinfection status and comorbid conditions in patients. New Microbes and New Infections. 2017;**20**:39-42

[20] Naqvi S, Bashir S, Rupareliya C, Shams A, Giyanwani PR, Ali Z, et al. Clinical spectrum of chikungunya in Pakistan. Cureus. 2017;**9**(7):e1430

[21] Manica M, Guzzetta G, Poletti P, Filipponi F, Solimini A, Caputo B, et al. Transmission dynamics of the ongoing chikungunya outbreak in Central Italy: From coastal areas to the metropolitan city of Rome, summer 2017. Bulletin Europeen sur les Maladies Transmissibles = European Communicable Disease Bulletin. Euro Surveillance. 2017;**22**(44):17-00685

[22] Furuya-Kanamori L, Liang S, Milinovich G, Magalhaes RJ, Clements AC, Hu W, et al. Co-distribution and co-infection of chikungunya and dengue viruses. BMC Infectious Diseases. 2016;**16**:84

[23] Waggoner JJ, Gresh L, Vargas MJ, et al. Viremia and clinical presentation in nicaraguan patients infected with Zika virus, chikungunya virus, and dengue virus. Clinical Infectious Diseases. 2016;**63**:1584

[24] Cleton N, Koopmansa M, Reimerinka J, Godekea G-J, Reusken C. Come fly with me: Review of clinically important arboviruses for global travelers. Journal of Clinical Virology. 2012;**55**(3):191-203

[25] Thiberville SD, Moyen N, Dupuis-Maguiraga L, Nougairede A, Gould EA, Roques P, et al. Chikungunya fever: Epidemiology, clinical syndrome, pathogenesis and therapy. Antiviral Research. 2013;**99**:345-370

[26] Schwartz O, Albert ML. Biology and pathogenesis of chikungunya virus. Nature Reviews. Microbiology. 2010;**8**(7):491-500

[27] Tsetsarkin KA, Vanlandingham DL, McGee CE, Higgs S. A single mutation in chikungunya virus affects vector specificity and epidemic potential. PLoS Pathogens. 2007;**3**:e201

[28] Nunes MRT, Faria NR, Vasconcelos JM, Golding N, Kraemer MUG, Oliveira LF, et al. Emergence and potential for spread of chikungunya virus in Brazil. BMC Medicine. 2015;**13**:102

[29] Volk SM, Chen R, Tsetsarkin KA, Adams AP, Garcia TI, Sall AA, et al. Genome-scale phylogenetic analyses of chikungunya virus reveal independent emergences of recent epidemics and various evolutionary rates. Journal of Virology. 2010;**84**:6497-6504

[30] Rougeron V, Sam IC, Caron M, Nkoghe D, Leroy E, Roques P. Chikungunya, a paradigm of neglected tropical disease that emerged to be a new health global risk. Journal of Clinical Virology. 2015;**64**:144-152

[31] Kautz TF, Díaz-González EE, Erasmus JH, Malo-García IR, Langsjoen RM,

Patterson EI, et al. Chikungunya virus as cause of febrile illness outbreak, Chiapas, Mexico, 2014. Emerging Infectious Diseases. 2015;**21**:2070-2073

[32] Sahadeo N, Mohammed H, Allicock OM, Auguste AJ, Widen SG, Badal K, et al. Molecular characterisation of chikungunya virus infections in Trinidad and comparison of clinical and laboratory features with dengue and other acute febrile cases. PLoS Neglected Tropical Diseases. 2015;**9**:e0004199

[33] Teixeira MJ, Andrade A, Costa MN, Castro J, Oliveira F, Goes CS, et al. East/Central/South/African genotype chikungunya virus, Brazil, 2014. Emerging Infectious Diseases. 2015;**21**(5):906-907

[34] Moyen N, Thiberville SD, Pastorino B, Nougairede A, Thirion L, Mombouli JV, et al. First reported chikungunya Fever outbreak in the republic of congo, 2011. PLoS One. 2014;**9**(12):e115938

[35] Demanou M, Sadeuh-Mba SA, Vanhecke C, Ndikweti R, Kouna TI, Inais NM, et al. Molecular characterization of chikungunya virus from three regions of Cameroon. Virologica Sinica. 2015;**30**(6):470-473

[36] Powers AM, Brault AC, Tesh RB, Weaver SC. Re-emergence of chikungunya and o'nyong-nyong viruses: Evidence for distinct geographical lineages and distant evolutionary relationships. The Journal of General Virology. 2000;**81**(Pt. 2):471-479

[37] Gérardin P, Barau G, Michault A, Bintner M, Randrianaivo H, Choker G, et al. Multidisciplinary prospective study of mother-to-child chikungunya virus infections on the island of La Réunion. PLoS Medicine. 2008;**5**:e60

[38] Simon F, Tolou H, Jeandel P. The unexpected chikungunya outbreak. La Revue de Médecine Interne. 2006;**27**:437-441

[39] Passi GR, Khan YZ, Chitnis DS. Chikungunya infection in neonates. Indian Pediatrics. 2008;**45**:240-242

[40] Gérardin P, Sampériz S, Ramful D, Boumahni B, Bintner M, Alessandri JL, et al. Neurocognitive outcome of children exposed to perinatal mother-to-child Chikungunya virus infection: the CHIMERE cohort study on Reunion Island. PLoS Neglected Tropical Diseases. 2014;**8**:e2996

[41] Burt FJ, Rolph MS, Rulli NE, Mahalingam S, Heise MT. Chikungunya: A re-emerging virus. Lancet. 2012;**379**:662-671

[42] Parola P, de Lamballerie X, Jourdan J, Rovery C, Vaillant V, Minodier P, et al. Novel chikungunya virus variant in travelers returning from Indian Ocean islands. Emerging Infectious Diseases. 2006;**12**:1493

[43] Taubitz W, Cramer JP, Kapaun A, Pfeffer M, Drosten C, Dobler G, et al. Chikungunya fever in travelers: Clinical presentation and course. Clinical Infectious Diseases. 2007;**45**:e1

[44] Simon F, Javelle E, Cabie A, Bouquillard E, Troisgros O, Gentile G, et al. French guidelines for the management of chikungunya (acute and persistent presentations). Médecine et Maladies Infectieuses. 2015;**45**(7):243-263

[45] Sissoko D, Malvy D, Ezzedine K, Renault P, Moscetti F, Ledrans M, et al. Post-epidemic chikungunya disease on Reunion Island: Course of rheumatic manifestations and associated factors over a 15-month period. PLoS Neglected Tropical Diseases. 2009;**3**(3):e389

[46] Chopra A, Anuradha V, Ghorpade R, Saluja M. Acute chikungunya and persistent musculoskeletal pain

following the 2006 Indian epidemic: A 2-year prospective rural community study. Epidemiology and Infection. 2012;**140**(5):842-850

[47] Edington F, Varjão D, Melo P. Incidence of articular pain and arthritis after chikungunya fever in the Americas: A systematic review of the literature and meta-analysis. Joint, Bone, Spine. 2018;**85**:669

[48] Haese NN, Broeckel RM, Hawman DW, et al. Animal models of chikungunya virus infection and disease. The Journal of Infectious Diseases. 2016;**214**(suppl_5):S482-S487

[49] Burt FJ, Chen W, Miner JJ, Lenschow DJ, Merits A, Schnettler E, et al. Chikungunya virus: An update on the biology and pathogenesis of this emerging pathogen. The Lancet Infectious Diseases. 2017;**17**(4):e107-e117

[50] Rodríguez-Morales AJ, Cardona-Ospina JA, Fernanda Urbano-Garzón S, Sebastian Hurtado-Zapata J. Prevalence of post-chikungunya infection chronic inflammatory arthritis: A systematic review and meta-analysis. Arthritis Care and Research. 2016;**68**(12):1849-1858

[51] Zaid A, Gérardin P, Taylor A, Mostafavi H, Malvy D, Mahalingam S. Chikungunya virus arthritis: Implications of acute and chronic inflammation mechanisms on patient management. Arthritis & Rhematology. 2018;**70**(4):484-495

[52] Marimoutou C, Ferraro J, Javelle E, Deparis X, Simon F. Chikungunya infection: Self-reported rheumatic morbidity and impaired quality of life persist 6 years later. Clinical Microbiology and Infection. 2015;**21**(7):688-693

[53] van Aalst M, Nelen CM, Goorhuis A, Stijnis C, Grobusch MP. Long-term sequelae of chikungunya virus disease: A systematic review. Travel Medicine and Infectious Disease. 2017;**15**:8-22

[54] Paixão ES, Rodrigues LC, Costa MDCN, Itaparica M, Barreto F, Gérardin P, et al. Chikungunya chronic disease: A systematic review and meta-analysis. Transactions of the Royal Society of Tropical Medicine and Hygiene. 2018;**112**(7):301-316

[55] Waymouth HE, Zoutman DE, Towheed TE. Chikungunya-related arthritis: Case report and review of the literature. Seminars in Arthritis and Rheumatism. 2013;**43**(2):273-278

[56] Chang LJ, Dowd KA, Mendoza FH, Saunders JG, Sitar S, Plummer SH, et al. Safety and tolerability of chikungunya virus-like particle vaccine in healthy adults: A phase 1 dose-escalation trial. Lancet. 2014;**384**:2046

[57] Ramsauer K, Schwameis M, Firbas C, Müllner M, Putnak RJ, Thomas SJ, et al. Immunogenicity, safety, and tolerability of a recombinant measles-virus-based chikungunya vaccine: A randomised, double-blind, placebo-controlled, active-comparator, first-in-man trial. The Lancet Infectious Diseases. 2015;**15**:519

[58] Reisinger EC, Tschismarov R, Beubler E, Wiedermann U, Firbas C, Loebermann M, et al. Immunogenicity, safety, and tolerability of the measles-vectored chikungunya virus vaccine MV-CHIK: A double-blind, randomised, placebo-controlled and active-controlled phase 2 trial. Lancet. 2019;**392**:2718

[59] Ribeiro AMBM, Pimentel CM, Guerra ACCG, Lima MRO. Physiotherapeutic approach on the late phase of chikungunya: A case report. Revista Brasileira de Saúde Materno Infantil. 2016;**16**(Suppl 1):S57-S62

[60] Bonifay T, Lienne JF, Bagoée C, Santa F, Vesin G, Walter G, et al. Prevalence and risk factors of post chikungunya rheumatic musculoskeletal disorders: A prospective follow-up study

in French Guiana. European Journal of Clinical Microbiology & Infectious Diseases. 2018;**37**(11):2159-2164

[61] CDC Press Releases [Internet]. CDC. 2016 [citado 10 de junio de 2019]. Disponible. https://www.cdc.gov/media/releases/2016/s0318-zika-lab-test.html

[62] Loconsole D, Metallo A, De Robertis AL, Morea A, Quarto M, Chironna M. Seroprevalence of dengue virus, West Nile virus, chikungunya virus, and Zika virus in International Travelers Attending a Travel and Migration Center in 2015-2017, Southern Italy. Vector Borne and Zoonotic Diseases. 2018;**18**(6):331-334

[63] Boga JA, Alvarez-Arguelles ME, Rojo-Alba S, Rodríguez M, de Oña M, Melón S. Simultaneous detection of dengue virus, chikungunya virus, Zika virus, yellow fever virus and West Nile virus. Journal of Virological Methods. 2019;**268**:53-55

[64] Pezzi L, Reusken CB, Weaver SC, Drexler JF, Busch M, LaBeaud D, et al. GloPID-R report on Chikungunya, O'nyong-nyong and Mayaro virus, part I: Biological diagnostics. Antiviral Research. 2019

[65] Lanciotti RS, Kosoy OL, Laven JJ, Panella AJ, Velez JO, Lambert AJ, et al. Chikungunya virus in US travelers returning from India, 2006. Emerging Infectious Diseases. 2007;**13**:764-767

[66] Chusri S, Siripaitoon P, Silpapojakul K, Hortiwakul T, Charernmak B, Chinnawirotpisan P, et al. Kinetics of chikungunya infections during an outbreak in Southern Thailand, 2008-2009. The American Journal of Tropical Medicine and Hygiene. 2014;**90**:410-417

[67] Beaty BJ, Calisher CH, Shope RE. Arboviruses. In: Lennette ELD, Lennette E, editors. Diagnostic Procedures for Viral, Rickettsial, and Chlamydial Infections. Washington, DC: American Public Health Association; 1995

[68] Martin DA, Muth DA, Brown T, Johnson AJ, Karabatsos N, Roehrig JT. Standardization of immunoglobulin M capture enzyme-linked immunosorbent assays for routine diagnosis of arboviral infections. Journal of Clinical Microbiology. 2000;**38**:1823-1826

[69] Martin DA, Noga A, Kosoy O, Johnson AJ, Petersen LR, Lanciotti RS. Evaluation of a diagnostic algorithm using immunoglobulin M enzyme-linked immunosorbent assay to differentiate human West Nile virus and St. Louis Encephalitis virus infections during the 2002 West Nile virus epidemic in the United States. Clinical and Diagnostic Laboratory Immunology. 2004;**11**:1130-1133

[70] Diagnostic Testing CDC [Internet]. 2018 [citado 10 de junio de 2019]. Disponible. https://www.cdc.gov/chikungunya/hc/diagnostic.html

[71] Lakshmi V, Neeraja M, Subbalaxmi MV, Parida MM, Dash PK, Santhosh SR, et al. Clinical features and molecular diagnosis of chikungunya fever from South India. Clinical Infectious Diseases. 2008;**46**:1436

[72] Panning M, Grywna K, van Esbroeck M, Emmerich P, Drosten C. Chikungunya fever in travelers returning to Europe from the Indian Ocean region, 2006. Emerging Infectious Diseases. 2008;**14**:416.9

[73] Simon F, Savini H, Parola P. Chikungunya: A paradigm of emergence and globalization of vector-borne diseases. The Medical Clinics of North America. 2008;**92**:1323

[74] Hussain KM, Lee RCH, Ng MM, Chu JJ. Establishment of a novel primary human skeletal myoblast cellular model for chikungunya virus infection and pathogenesis. Scientific Reports. 2016;**6**:21406

[75] Her Z, Malleret B, Chan M, Ong EK, Wong SC, Kwek DJ, et al. Active infection of human blood monocytes by chikungunyavirustriggers an innate immune response. Journal of Immunology. 2010;**184**:5903-5913

[76] Parashar D, Paingankar MS, Kumar S, Gokhale MD, Sudeep AB, Shinde SB, et al. Administration of E2 and NS1 siRNAs inhibit chikungunya virus replication in vitro and protects mice infected with the virus. PLoS Neglected Tropical Diseases. 2013;**7**:e2405

[77] Phuklia W, Kasisith J, Modhiran N, Rodpai E, Thannagith M, Thongsakulprasert T, et al. Osteoclastogenesis induced by CHIKV-infected fibroblast-like synoviocytes: A possible interplay between synoviocytes and monocytes/macrophages in CHIKV-induced arthralgia/arthritis. Virus Research. 2013;**177**:179-188

[78] Pyndiah MN, Pursem V, Meetoo G, Daby S, Ramuth V, Bhinkah P, et al. Chikungunya virus isolation using simplified cell culture technique in Mauritius. Medecine Tropicale (Mars). 2012;**72**:63-65

[79] Jain J, Okabayashi T, Kaur N, Nakayama E, Shioda T, Gaind R, et al. Evaluation of an immunochro matography rapid diagnosis kit for detection of chikungunya virus antigen in India, a dengue-endemic country. Virology Journal. 2018;**15**:84

[80] Okabayashi T, Sasaki T, Masrinoul P, Chantawat N, Yoksan S, Nitatpattana N, et al. Detection of chikungunya virus antigen by a novel rapid immunochromatographic test. Journal of Clinical Microbiology. 2015;**53**:382e8

[81] de Morais Bronzoni RV, Baleotti FG, Ribeiro Nogueira RM, Nunes M, Moraes Figueiredo LT. Duplex reverse transcription-PCR followed by nested PCR assays for detection and identification of Brazilian alphaviruses and flaviviruses. Journal of Clinical Microbiology. 2005;**43**(2):696-702

[82] Carletti F, Bordi L, Chiappini R, Ippolito G, Sciarrone MR, Capobianchi MR, et al. Rapid detection and quantification of Chikungunya virus by a one-step reverse transcription polymerase chain reaction real-time assay. American Journal of Tropical Medicine and Hygiene. 2007;**77**(3):521-524. 12, 14

[83] Pastorino B, Bessaud M, Grandadam M, Murri S, Murri S, Tolou HJ, et al. Development of a TaqMan RT-PCR assay without RNA extraction step for the detection and quantification of African chikungunya viruses. Journal of Virological Methods. 2005;**124**:65-71

[84] Edwards CJ, Welch SR, Chamberlain J, Hewson R, Tolley H, Cane PA, et al. Molecular diagnosis and analysis of chikungunya virus. Journal of Clinical Virology. 2007;**39**:271-275

[85] Parida MM, Santhosh SR, Dash PK, Tripathi NK, Lakshmi V, Mamidi N, et al. Rapid and real-time detection of chikungunya virus by reverse transcription loop-mediated isothermal amplification assay. Journal of Clinical Microbiology. 2007;**45**:351-357

[86] Panning M, Hess M, Fischer W, Grywna K, Grywna K, Pfeffer M, et al. Performance of the RealStar chikungunya virus real-time reverse transcription-PCR kit. Journal of Clinical Microbiology. 2009;**47**:3014-3016

[87] Ho PS, Ng MM, Chu JJ. Establishment of one-step SYBR green-based real time-PCR assay for rapid detection and quantification of chikungunya virus infection. Virology Journal. 2010;**7**:13

[88] Ummul Haninah A, Vasan SS, Ravindran T, Chandru A, Lee HL,

Shamala Devi S. Development and evaluation of a one-step SYBR-Green I-based real-time RT-PCR assay for the detection and quantification of chikungunya virus in human, monkey and mosquito samples. Tropical Biomedicine. 2010;**27**:611-623

[89] Plaskon NE, Adelman ZN, Myles KM. Accurate strand-specific quantification of viral RNA. PLoS One. 2009;**4**:e7468

[90] Chiam CW, Chan YF, Loong SK, Yong SS, Yong SS, Hooi PS, et al. Real-time polymerase chain reaction for diagnosis and quantitation of negative strand of chikungunya virus. Diagnostic Microbiology and Infectious Disease. 2013;**77**:133-137

[91] Parida MM, Santhosh SR, Dash PK, Lakshmana Rao PV. Rapid and real-time assays for detection and quantification of chikungunya virus. Future Virology. 2008;**3**:179-192

[92] Reddy V, Ravi V, Desai A, Parida M, Powers AM, Johnson BW. Utility of IgM ELISA, TaqMan real-time PCR, reverse transcription PCR, and RT-LAMP assay for the diagnosis of chikungunya fever. Journal of Medical Virology. 2012;**84**:1771-1778

[93] Tan JL, Capozzoli M, Mitsuharu S, Watthanaworawit W, Ling CL, Mauduit M, et al. An integrated lab-on-chip for rapid identification and simultaneous differentiation of tropical pathogens. PLoS Neglected Tropical Diseases. 2014;**8**:e3043

[94] Lanciotti RS, Valadere AM. Transcontinental movement of Asian genotype chikungunya virus. Emerging Infectious Diseases. 2014;**20**:1400-1402

[95] Lanciotti RS, Lambert AJ. Phylogenetic analysis of chikungunya virus strains circulating in the Western Hemisphere. The American Journal of Tropical Medicine and Hygiene. 2016;**94**:800-803

[96] Santhosh SR, Dash PK, Parida M, Khan M, Rao PV. Appearance of E1: A226V mutant chikungunya virus in Coastal Karnataka, India during 2008 outbreak. Virology Journal. 2009;**6**:172. DOI: 10.1186/1743-422X-6-172

[97] Niyas KP, Abraham R, Unnikrishnan RN, Mathew T, Nair S, Manakkadan A, et al. Molecular characterization of Chikungunya virus isolates from clinical samples and adult Aedes albopictus mosquitoes emerged from larvae from Kerala, South India. Virology Journal. 2010;**7**(1):189

[98] Kucharz EJ, Cebula-Byrska I. Chikungunya fever. European Journal of Internal Medicine. 2014;**23**:325-329

[99] Prat CM, Flusin O, Panella A, Tenebray B, Lanciotti R, Leparc-Goffart I. Evaluation of commercially available serologic diagnostic tests for Chikungunya virus. Emerging Infectious Diseases. 2014;**20**:2129-2132

[100] Yap G, Pok KY, Lai YL, Hapuarachchi HC, Chow A, Leo YS, et al. Evaluation of chikungunya diagnostic assays: Differences in sensitivity of serology assays in two independent outbreaks. PLoS Neglected Tropical Diseases. 2014;**4**:e753

[101] LaBeaud AD, Banda T, Brichard J, Muchiri EM, Mungai PL, Mutuku FM, et al. High rates of o'nyongnyong and chikungunya virus transmission in coastal Kenya. PLoS Neglected Tropical Diseases. 2015;**9**:e0003436

[102] Cavrini F, Gaibani P, Pierro AM, Rossini G, Landini MP, Sambri V. Chikungunya: An emerging and spreading arthropod-borne viral disease. Journal of Infection in Developing Countries. 2009;**3**:744-752

[103] Pialoux G, Gaüzère BA, Jauréguiberry S, Strobel M. Chikungunya, an epidemic arbovirosis. The Lancet Infectious Diseases. 2007;7:319-327

[104] Blacksell SD, Tanganuchitcharnchai A, Jarman RG, Gibbons RV, Paris DH, Bailey MS, et al. Poor diagnostic accuracy of commercial antibody-based assays for the diagnosis of acute chikungunya infection. Clinical and Vaccine Immunology. 2011;**18**:1773-1775

[105] Rianthavorn P, Wuttirattanakowit N, Prianantathavorn K, Limpaphayom N, Theamboonlers A, Poovorawan Y. Evaluation of a rapid assay for detection of IgM antibodies to chikungunya. The Southeast Asian Journal of Tropical Medicine and Public Health. 2010;**41**(1):92-96

[106] Yap G, Pok KY, Lai YL, Hapuarachchi HC, Chow A, Leo YS, et al. Evaluation of chikungunya diagnostic assays: Differences in sensitivity of serology assays in two independent outbreaks. PLoS Neglected Tropical Diseases. 2010;**4**:e753

[107] Sambri V, Capobianchi MR, Cavrini F, Charrel R, Donoso-Mantke O, Escadafal C, et al. Diagnosis of West Nile virus human infections: Overview and proposal of diagnostic protocols considering the results of external quality assessment studies. Viruses. 2013;**5**:2329-2348

[108] Brouard C, Bernillon P, Quatresous I, Pillonel J, Assal A, De Valk H, et al. Estimated risk of chikungunya viremic blood donation during an epidemic on Reunion Island in the Indian Ocean, 2005 to 2007. Transfusion. 2008;**48**:1333

[109] Simmons G, Brès V, Lu K, Liss NM, Brambilla DJ, Ryff KR, et al. High incidence of chikungunya virus and frequency of viremic blood donations during epidemic, Puerto Rico, USA, 2014. Emerging Infectious Diseases. 2016;**22**:1221

[110] Rosso F, Rodríguez S, Cedano JA, Mora BL, Moncada PA, Velez JD. Chikungunya in solid organ transplant recipients, a case series and literature review. Transplant Infectious Disease. 2018;**20**(6):e1297

[111] Touret Y, Randrianaivo H, Michault A, Schuffenecker I, Kauffmann E, Lenglet Y, et al. Early maternal-fetal transmission of the chikungunya virus. Presse Médicale. 2006;**35**:1656-1658

[112] Robillard PY, Boumahni B, Gérardin P, Michault A, Fourmaintraux A, Schuffenecker I, et al. Vertical maternal fetal transmission of the chikungunya virus: Ten cases among 84 pregnant women. Presse Médicale. 2006;**35**:785-788

[113] Torres JR, Falleiros-Arlant LH, Dueñas L, Pleitez-Navarrete J, Salgado DM, Castillo JB. Congenital and perinatal complications of chikungunya fever: A Latin American experience. International Journal of Infectious Diseases. 2016;**51**:85-88

[114] Fritel X, Catteau C, Calliez F, Brodel A, Vaillant JL, Ansquin H. Chikungunya outbreak, pregnancy outcome and perinatal mortality: Observational study about 40,000 pregnancies and deliveries on Réunion island, during 2004-2006. In: Proceedings of the 13th International Congress on Infectious Disease, 2008 June 19-22, Kuala Lumpur. Abstract published in: Int J Infect Dis. Vol. 12, No. Suppl 1. 2008. p. e328

[115] Fritel X, Rollot O, Gérardin P, Gauzere BA, Bideault J, Lagarde L, et al. Chikungunya virus infection

during pregnancy, Reunion, France, 2006. Emerging Infectious Diseases. 2010;**16**:418-425

[116] Gérardin P, LaBeaud AD, Ritz N. Chikungunya fever during pregnancy and in children: and overview on clinical and research perspectives. Intech Open Access. 2016. p. 19-41. DOI: 10.5772/64424

[117] Barr KL. Vaidhyanathan V, Chikungunya in infants and children: Is pathogenesis increasing? Viruses. 2019;**11**(3):23

[118] Lewthwaite P, Vasanthapuram R, Osborne JC, Begum A, Plank JL, Shankar MV, et al. Chikungunya virus and central nervous system infections in children, India. Emerging Infectious Diseases. 2009;**15**:329-331

[119] Ramful D, Carbonnier M, Pasquet M, Bouhmani B, Ghazouani J, Noormahomed T, et al. Mother-to-child transmission of chikungunya virus infection. The Pediatric Infectious Disease Journal. 2007;**26**:811-815

[120] Maron BJ, Tajik AJ, Ruttenberg HD, Graham TP, Atwood GF, Victorica BE, et al. Hypertrophic cardiomyopathy in infants: Mother-to-child transmission of chikungunya. Circulation. 1982;**65**:7-17

[121] Sewell EK, Keene S. Perinatal care of infants with congenital birth defects. Clinics in Perinatology. 2018;**45**:213-230

[122] Schuffenecker I, Iteman I, Michault A, Murri S, Frangeul L, Vaney MC, et al. Genome microevolution of chikungunya viruses causing the Indian ocean outbreak. PLoS Medicine. 2006;**3**:e263

[123] Jadhav M, Namboodripad M, Carman RH, Carey DE, Myers RM. Chikungunya disease in infants and children in Vellore: A report of clinical and haematological features of virologically proved cases. The Indian Journal of Medical Research. 1965;**53**:764-776

[124] Vu-Qui-Dai, Nguyen-Thi Kim-Thoa, Ly-Quoc-Bang. Study of anti-chikungunya antibodies in Vietnamese children in Saigon. Bulletin de la Societe de Pathologie Exotique et de Ses Filiales. 1967;**60**:353-359

[125] Carey DE, Myers RM, DeRanitz CM, Jadhav M, Reuben R. The 1964 chikungunya epidemic at Vellore, South India, including observations on concurrent dengue. Transactions of the Royal Society of Tropical Medicine and Hygiene. 1969;**63**:434-445

[126] Halstead SB, Udomsakdi S, Singharaj P, Nisalak A. Dengue chikungunya virus infection in man in Thailand, 1962-1964. 3. Clinical, epidemiologic, and virologic observations on disease in non-indigenous white persons. The American Journal of Tropical Medicine and Hygiene. 1969;**18**:984-996

[127] Nimmannitya S, Halstead SB, Cohen SN, Margiotta M. Dengue and chikungunya virus infection in man in Thailand, 1962-1964. I. Observations on hospitalized patients with hemorrhagic fever. The American Journal of Tropical Medicine and Hygiene. 1969;**18**:954-971

Chapter 4

Clinical Features and Management of Chronic Chikungunya Arthritis

Joshua Britton Bilsborrow, José Kennedy Amaral and Robert T. Schoen

Abstract

Chikungunya virus is a single-stranded RNA alphavirus transmitted to humans by *Aedes* species mosquitos, causing an acute illness known as chikungunya fever with maculopapular rash, headache, polyarthritis/arthralgias, and gastrointestinal symptoms. Up to half of affected patients develop a chronic disabling arthritis following resolution of the acute infection, which can last for months or even years. The pathophysiology of chronic chikungunya arthritis remains controversial; it may result from a dysregulated immune response or be caused by persistent viral infection. Treatment for patients with chronic chikungunya arthritis remains investigational. Limited data suggests that immunosuppressive therapies such as methotrexate and TNF alpha inhibitors may be beneficial, though randomized clinical trials are needed.

Keywords: chikungunya, alphavirus, arthritis, disability, DMARDs

1. Introduction

Chikungunya virus (CHIKV) is a small, single-stranded RNA alphavirus transmitted to humans by *Aedes* species mosquitoes, including *Aedes aegypti* and *Aedes albopictus*. CHIKV was initially isolated in Tanzania in 1952–1953 [1]. The word "chikungunya" means "that which bends up" or "to become contorted" in the Makonde language, referring to the prostrated appearance of affected patients [2].

Prior to its isolation, chikungunya (CHIK) was often misdiagnosed as dengue [3]. During the twentieth century, chikungunya fever (CHIKF) epidemics occurred sporadically and were limited to Africa and Asia, but in the twenty-first century CHIK has become a global disease. There was a major outbreak in coastal Kenya in 2004, which subsequently spread to Réunion in 2005 and throughout the Indian Ocean region [4]. Cases among travelers returning from endemic regions were reported in Italy in 2007 [5].

CHIKV reached the Western Hemisphere in 2013 with an outbreak on the island of Saint Martin. Since then, the virus has spread throughout the region with more than 2 million cases documented in the Americas by the end of 2016, though the actual number is likely much higher [3]. In the United States, cases involving travelers to endemic regions have been documented in 49 states, and locally-acquired cases have occurred in Florida and Texas [6].

Factors contributing to the spread of CHIK include increasing urbanization, overstrained health care infrastructures in developing countries, ease of international travel, and climate change with expansion of mosquito vectors [7].

There are three known genotypes of CHIKV: Asia, East/Central/South Africa, and West Africa. The 2004–2005 pandemic that originated in Kenya and subsequently spread throughout the Indian Ocean region involved the East/Central/South Africa genotype. The pandemic that emerged in the Americas in 2013 originally involved the Asia genotype, although more recently the East/Central/South Africa lineage has been reported in the Western Hemisphere [8, 9].

2. Clinical manifestations

2.1 Acute chikungunya fever

CHIKV infection results from transmission by the mosquito vector. Following an incubation period of 5–7 days, patients develop an acute febrile illness, chikungunya fever (CHIKF), characterized by high fevers, maculopapular rash, headaches, polyarthritis/arthralgias, myalgias, nausea, vomiting, and diarrhea [1]. Joint pain is often severe, and most often involves the metacarpal-phalangeal and interphalangeal joints of the hands, the wrists, the ankles, and the metatarsal-phalangeal joints of the feet. Less commonly involved but described joints include the shoulders, elbows, hips, knees, and inter-vertebral joints [10]. Acute CHIKF causes significant physical disability. For example, during the 2005 Comoros epidemic, an estimated 80% of affected patients were hospitalized or bed-bound due to severity of their symptoms [11].

More severely affected patients can develop neurological disease including meningoencephalitis, myelitis, radiculitis, and/or peripheral neuropathy, including reports of Guillain-Barré syndrome [12]. Rare ophthalmological manifestations reported include keratitis, episcleritis, optic neuritis, uveitis, and retinal detachment [13]. Uncommon but serious cardiac manifestations include arrhythmias, vasculopathy, myocarditis, and/or dilated cardiomyopathy [14, 15]. Patients with acute infection can have laboratory abnormalities including thrombocytopenia and leukopenia (lymphopenia is more common than neutropenia) [4].

Maternal-to-child transmission has also been reported, with up to 50% of neonates acquiring infection during childbirth if born within 5 days of maternal infection. Musculoskeletal manifestations are less prominent in newborns, with CHIKF being more notable for fevers, rash, cytopenias, hepatitis, and/or encephalitis [16].

Acute CHIKF typically resolves in 10–14 days, and has an overall reported case fatality rate of <1% based on epidemics in the Indian Ocean region and the Americas. However, the case fatality rate is higher among newborns, the elderly, and patients with underlying cardiovascular and pulmonary conditions [7, 17, 18]. Economopoulou and colleagues studied the case fatality rate among atypical cases of CHIKF in Réunion (defined as patients presenting with symptoms other than fevers and arthralgias); 65/610 patients from this group died for a case fatality rate of 10.6% [19].

During the widespread Indian Ocean region pandemic, a point mutation (A226V) in the E1 surface glycoprotein of CHIKV may have allowed better adaptation in *Aedes albopictus*, which had previously been a minor vector [20]. Along with low background immunity among populations residing in regions not historically affected, this may account for the rapid spread and high rates of infectivity seen for CHIKV in the twenty-first century.

2.2 Chronic chikungunya arthritis

Arthritis/arthralgia is a principal feature of CHIKF. Many patients recover within several weeks, but up to 50% develop chronic joint pain and swelling. When rheumatic disease persists for more than 12 weeks, we refer to these symptoms as chronic chikungunya arthritis (CCA). Arthritic manifestations can last for weeks, months, or even years [21]. Rodriguez-Morales and colleagues retrospectively studied 283 patients from the 2015 epidemic in Risaralda Department, Colombia. At 26 weeks post-infection, 53.7% of the patients reported chronic musculoskeletal symptoms, including 49.5% with morning stiffness, 40.6% with joint swelling, and 16.6% with joint erythema [22]. Another large observational study from Kerala, India found that 57% of patients had chronic polyarthralgias, 22% chronic polyarthritis, and 19.5% chronic tenosynovitis 15 months after CHIKF [23].

The classical pattern of arthritis involves the small-to-medium sized joints in a peripheral and symmetric distribution [24]. This pattern can resemble rheumatoid arthritis (RA). Joint pain with/without synovitis can persist following acute CHIKF, or joint symptoms may remit and then recur at a later time [21].

A prospective Mexican cohort study showed that greater severity of acute infection predicted development of chronic arthritis, as measured by the disease activity index 28 (DAS28), World Health Organization Disablement Assessment Schedule II (WHODAS-II), and serum IL-6 level [25]. Other risk factors for chronic disease include patient age >45 years and high viral load ($>10^9$ per ml) during acute infection [26].

During acute CHIK infection, serum cytokines IL-1Ra, IL-1β, IL-6, IL-7, IL-8, IL-12, IL-15, and IFN-α increase, while RANTES (CCL5) decreases [27, 28]. With the transition to CCA, elevated levels of IL-6, GM-CSF, and IL-17 become predominant [28]. The IL-17 signature in particular may drive chronic joint inflammation, stimulating the upregulation of other pro-inflammatory cytokines, including IL-1, IL-6, and TNF-α, matrix metalloproteinases, and RANK-RANKL leading to osteoclastogenesis and bone erosions [29]. Alphavirus infection of osteoblasts has been shown to perturb the RANKL-osteoprotegerin ratio, contributing to bone loss. This imbalance may also provide a mechanism for joint erosions in chronic disease [30].

CHIKV primarily infects human epithelial and endothelial cells, fibroblasts, and macrophages. Replication has not been observed in lymphocytes, monocytes, or monocyte-derived dendritic cells [31]. Viral tropism to the highly-vascularized synovial tissues of the joints may be responsible for the prominence of arthritis following acute infection. Whether CHIKV persists in synovial tissue during the chronic phase remains unclear, however, and there is ongoing debate about whether CCA arises secondary to immunological dysregulation or is due to persistent alphavirus infection of the synovial tissue.

Hoarau and colleagues demonstrated the presence of CHIKV RNA and viral proteins within perivascular synovial macrophages from one patient with CCA 18 months following acute infection [32]. This finding has not been replicated in other patients with chronic joint disease, however. Viral RNA has been isolated from knee synovial tissue of patients infected with a related alphavirus, Ross River virus [33]. In non-human primates, CHIKV can be recovered from muscle, synovial, lymphoid, and hepatic tissues following resolution of acute infection. Macrophages have also been identified as viral reservoirs [34].

In a cohort from the Réunion epidemic, 16 CCA patients were evaluated for persistence of viral infection. Synovial fluid (10 patients) and biopsied tissue (6 patients) was evaluated with reverse transcriptase polymerase chain reaction (RT-PCR) for CHIKV. All samples were negative, suggesting active viral replication is not the cause of chronic articular disease [35].

These findings were replicated in a Colombian cohort with CCA, evaluated during the 2014–2015 epidemic. In all patients, synovial fluid was aspirated from inflamed joints. CHIKV DNA was not recovered by RT-PCR, viral proteins were not detected by mass spectrometry, and viral cultures were also negative for all patients. The authors concluded that CCA is probably a post-infectious autoimmune process [36].

Evidence for molecular mimicry between host tissues and CHIKV E1 glycoprotein has been postulated [37]. However, the specific mechanisms by which CHIK infection might lead to immunological dysregulation and autoimmunity are unknown.

2.3 Diagnosis of chronic chikungunya arthritis

The diagnosis of CHIK depends on epidemiologic information, characteristic clinical features, the time course of the infection, and laboratory confirmation. Many patients live in or have had recent travel to an area with endemic transmission of *Aedes* mosquitos. Laboratory testing depends on the time course of infection. During acute disease, CHIK viremia lasts for 5–7 days. At this time, RT-PCR of serum can be diagnostic. Anti-CHIKV IgM antibodies appear at 3–8 days and remain positive for 1–3 months. Anti-CHIKV IgG antibodies are detectable at 4–10 days and remain positive for months to years [1].

CCA patients present with chronic debilitating joint symptoms ranging from morning stiffness and arthralgias to frank inflammatory synovitis. A classical pattern of small-and-medium joint peripheral involvement has been described, but mono- and oligoarthritis can also occur (**Figure 1**). In some patients, CCA presents clinically as an RA "mimic," but most patients have negative tests for rheumatoid factor and anti-cyclic citrullinated peptide antibodies [38]. Patients with CCA often meet diagnostic and/or clinical criteria for RA or spondyloarthritis [39]. The distinguishing clinical feature is a previous history of acute CHIKF, with laboratory confirmation of serum positivity for IgM and/or IgG anti-CHIK antibodies.

Radiographic imaging of involved joints may be normal, especially early in the disease, with progression to bone erosions in some patients over time. Magnetic resonance imaging has greater sensitivity for the detection of inflammatory changes, and can show synovial thickening, bone marrow edema, effusions, and/or tenosynovitis [38].

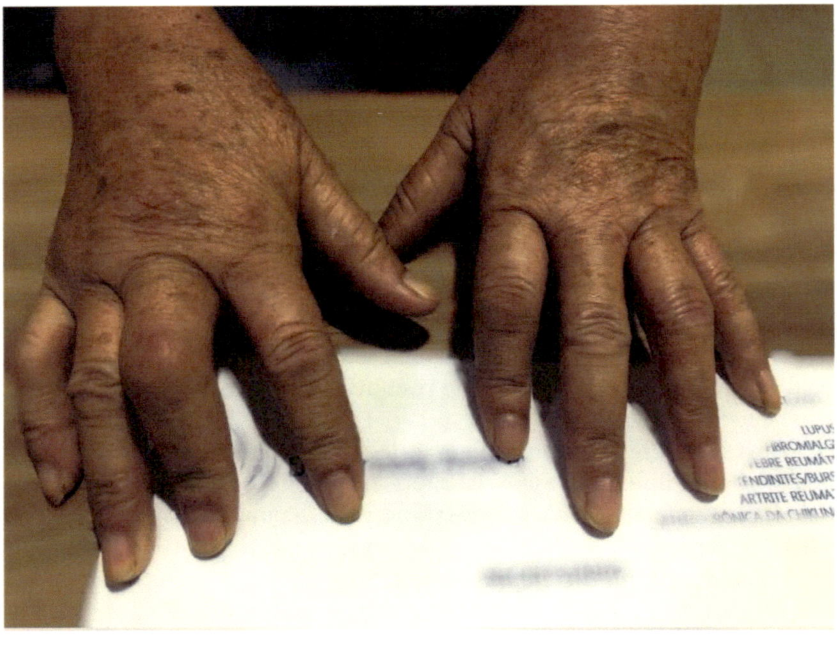

Figure 1.
Patient with chronic chikungunya arthritis (CCA). A 50-year-old woman with CCA and synovitis of the right third PIP and left second PIP joints. She had acute CHIKF 3 years prior and subsequently developed CCA of the hand joints. Image courtesy of José Kennedy Amaral, M.D., Pernambuco, Brazil.

3. Treatment of chronic chikungunya arthritis

Guidelines for the management of CCA emphasize symptomatic pain control with acetaminophen/paracetamol, codeine, and/or neuropathic medications such as gabapentin. Adjunctive treatment includes physical therapy, thermotherapy, and/or cryotherapy [16]. These approaches can relieve pain and improve function, but are not disease-modifying.

3.1 Corticosteroids and non-steroidal anti-inflammatory drugs (NSAIDs)

In an uncontrolled case series during the 2005–2006 Indian Ocean pandemic, short-term corticosteroid treatment improved arthritis and tenosynovitis, and reduced disability in patients with CCA [40]. Corticosteroid treatment led to greater pain relief and patient satisfaction compared to paracetamol, NSAIDs, medicinal herbs, and physical exercise [41].

Padmakumar and colleagues performed a randomized-controlled trial evaluating the efficacy of single and combination NSAID and corticosteroid treatment regimens for CCA. Functional and pain assessments improved with corticosteroids (prednisolone 10 mg daily) in addition to the NSAID aceclofenac 200 mg daily, compared to those who received aceclofenac alone. The addition of hydroxychloroquine (HCQ) did not provide added benefit [42].

Despite positive results, long-term use of corticosteroids is not advised due to well-known risks of infection, cataracts, glaucoma, hyperglycemia and diabetes mellitus, and osteopenia/osteoporosis associated with chronic corticosteroid use.

3.2 Chloroquine and hydroxychloroquine

An open-label pilot study of chloroquine (CQ) treatment for CCA in South Africa showed improvement in patient and physician disease activity assessments, though this trial was not blinded [43]. Brito and colleagues recommended HCQ at a dose of 6 mg/kg daily as first-line treatment for CCA, as part of a regimen potentially escalating to triple therapy with sulfasalazine (SSZ) and methotrexate (MTX) [44].

However, a randomized-controlled trial comparing short-term treatment with CQ to placebo for acute CHIK arthritis found no differences between-group in the duration of arthralgias or viremia, but increased rates of chronic arthralgias in the treated group [45]. Chopra and colleagues performed a comparative effectiveness trial between CQ 250 mg daily and meloxicam 7.5 mg daily in patients with CCA and found no difference in efficacy [46].

In the open-label randomized trial by Ravindran and Alias, combination therapy (MTX 15 mg weekly, SSZ 1000 mg daily, and HCQ 400 mg daily) was superior to HCQ monotherapy [47]. The trial did not include a placebo group, precluding the possibility of determining the efficacy of HCQ.

Overall, most current evidence suggests that antimalarials such as CQ and HCQ are not effective for the treatment of CCA.

3.3 Sulfasalazine

The Ravindran and Alias trial included SSZ 1000 mg daily in combination with HCQ and MTX as part of triple therapy, compared to HCQ [47]. While combination therapy was more efficacious, the contribution of SSZ separate from MTX could not be established.

Ganu and Ganu evaluated a cohort of 16 patients with persistent arthritis following acute CHIKF, comparing treatment with SSZ and MTX to SSZ alone. Improvement was noted in 71.4% of patients receiving combination therapy compared to 12.5% of patients receiving SSZ monotherapy [48]. A significant limitation of this trial was the lack of a control group; it remains questionable whether SSZ was any more effective than a placebo response. In addition, a majority of the patients had anti-cyclic citrullinated peptide antibodies, suggesting they had RA rather than CCA.

Overall, there is very limited data suggesting efficacy of SSZ monotherapy for the treatment of CCA, but it may be efficacious in combination with other medications such as MTX.

3.4 Methotrexate

Pandya treated 149 Indian patients with CCA with MTX 15–20 mg weekly in combination with HCQ. At 16 weeks, ACR20 responses were achieved in 48.9%, ACR50 in 18.8%, and ACR70 in 4.0%. Clinical response was less robust as measured by DAS28-ESR, with just 1/149 patients achieving clinical remission (DAS28-ESR <2.6) and only 4/149 with a good clinical response (DAS28-ESR <3.2) [49]. One important limitation of the study was that the diagnosis of CCA was made entirely on clinical grounds, without serological confirmation of anti-CHIKV antibodies. As such, the patient population may have been heterogeneous, including non-CHIK inflammatory arthritis syndromes.

In the trial by Ravindran and Alias, the combination therapy regimen including MTX 15 mg weekly (along with SSZ 1000 mg daily and HCQ 400 mg daily) was superior to HCQ alone (DAS28-ESR <3.2 at 24 weeks, 84% versus 14% respectively). Both groups also received prednisolone 7.5 mg daily, but this was tapered off by 6 weeks [47]. In another trial by Ganu and Ganu, patients with an inadequate treatment response to combination SSZ and HCQ were escalated to treatment with MTX 15–20 mg weekly versus placebo. The MTX group achieved a superior clinical response versus SSZ/HCQ (71.4% versus 12.5%) [48].

Javelle and colleagues reported on treatment of a Réunion cohort with CCA following the 2005-2006 epidemic. Among patients treated with MTX 7.5–25 mg weekly, 54/72 (75%) achieved a good clinical response [39].

Bouquillard and Combe treated patients with acute CHIKF who were subsequently diagnosed with RA. Among 19 patients treated with MTX, 13 had a good clinical response (68.4%). Among these patients, 54.1% were positive for rheumatoid factor, and 28.6% had anti-cyclic citrullinated peptide antibodies [50]. As such, many of the patients were diagnosed with seronegative RA, which can closely mimic the signs and symptoms of CCA, and which might respond to similar treatments.

Amaral and colleagues treated 48 patients with CCA with open-label MTX initiated at 7.5 mg weekly, with dose escalations for refractory symptoms at 4 weeks. The final mean MTX dose was 9.2 ± 3.2 mg per week. MTX therapy was combined with prednisone at a mean daily dose of 6.1 ± 2.2 mg for nine patients (18%). Two patients received HCQ (400 mg daily) with MTX, and one also received SSZ (1000 mg daily). At the first visit, the mean value for pain by visual analog scale was 7.7 ± 2.0. The mean values for pain at 4 and 8 weeks, compared to baseline, decreased to 3.0 and 2.6 respectively [24].

Overall, MTX has shown promise in the treatment of CCA, though previous trials have either combined MTX with HCQ and SSZ, or have been unblinded. Further randomized trials are needed to evaluate MTX monotherapy.

3.5 Biologics

No human trials have yet been conducted to evaluate the efficacy of biologic therapy with monoclonal antibodies for the treatment of CCA.

Ross River virus (RRV) is an alphavirus phylogenetically related to CHIKV. In RRV infected mice, treatment with the TNF-α inhibitor etanercept resulted in decreased weight gain, increased viral titers, and increased inflammatory cell recruitment and tissue damage [51]. This study suggests that etanercept treatment of human patients with acute CHIKF might be detrimental, though treatment of patients with CCA could have a different outcome.

Bouquillard and Combe treated patients with acute CHIKF followed by the diagnosis of RA (not categorized as CCA) with TNF-α inhibitors. These patients had been refractory to initial therapy with MTX. 6/6 patients had a good clinical response (four with etanercept, two with adalimumab) [50]. The majority of the patients had been diagnosed with seronegative RA, which was not distinguished from CCA.

Treatment of CHIKV acutely-infected mice with the anti-CTLA-4 monoclonal antibody abatacept showed decreased T cell infiltration of joint tissues without affecting viral replication [52]. There is currently no data for its use in humans, nor for its use in treating CCA.

3.6 Novel agents

Pentosan polysulfate is a novel glycosaminoglycan-like molecule developed for the treatment of alphavirus infections. Treatment of CHIKV-infected mice with pentosan polysulfate reduced cartilage thinning and immunological infiltration of joints [53]. Intra-articular levels of the pro-inflammatory cytokines IL-6, IL-9, CCL2, and G-CSF were decreased, and levels of the anti-inflammatory IL-10 were increased through unclear mechanisms [30]. While developed for the treatment of acute CHIK infection, it remains unclear if pentosan polysulfate could be used for the treatment of CCA, in particular to prevent joint erosions.

Fingolimod is a sphingosine 1-phosphate receptor agonist developed for the treatment of multiple sclerosis. In CHIKV-infected mice, fingolimod treatment decreased the migration of CD4+ T cells into joints without affecting viral replication [54]. While the utility of fingolimod for treatment of CCA remains unknown, decreasing T cell migration into joints might be beneficial.

4. Conclusions

CCA is an emerging chronic and disabling rheumatological syndrome which can persist for weeks, months, or years after acute CHIKF. With the global spread of CHIKV in past decades, increasing numbers of patients from developing countries in particular have acquired or are at risk for this chronic disabling rheumatic syndrome.

The pathophysiology of the disease remains uncertain, though the weight of evidence suggests that the syndrome is caused by a post-viral autoimmune process, which follows viral clearance.

There is limited clinical trial evidence for the use of disease modifying therapeutics for patients with CCA. Most previous trials have been open-label or of limited quality. Empiric treatment courses with corticosteroids, NSAIDs, antimalarials, and SSZ can be considered. However, given similarities between CCA and RA, it is our opinion that management with MTX should be further evaluated. Over time, new treatments including biologics and novel agents (pentosan polysulfate, fingolimod) may also emerge as treatment options.

Conflicts of interest

None of the authors have any conflicts of interest to report.

Funding source

None.

Author details

Joshua Britton Bilsborrow[1], José Kennedy Amaral[2] and Robert T. Schoen[1*]

1 Section of Rheumatology, Allergy and Immunology, Yale University School of Medicine, New Haven, Connecticut, United States of America

2 Department of Infectious Diseases and Tropical Medicine, Federal University of Minas Gerais, Belo Horizonte, Minas Gerais, Brazil

*Address all correspondence to: robert.schoen@yale.edu

References

[1] Suhrbier A, Jaffar-Bandjee MC, Gasque P. Arthritogenic alphaviruses: An overview. Nature Reviews Rheumatology. 2012;**8**(7):420-429

[2] Ganesan VK, Duan B, Reid SP. Chikungunya virus: Pathophysiology, mechanism, and modeling. Viruses. 2017;**9**(12):368

[3] Silva LA, Dermody TS. Chikungunya virus: Epidemiology, replication, disease mechanisms, and prospective intervention strategies. The Journal of Clinical Investigation. 2017;**127**(3):737-749

[4] Staples JE, Breiman RF, Powers AM. Chikungunya fever: An epidemiological review of a re-emerging infectious disease. Clinical Infectious Diseases. 2009;**49**(6):942-948

[5] Rezza G. Chikungunya is back in Italy: 2007-2017. Journal of Travel Medicine. 2018;**25**(1). DOI: 10.1093/jtm/tay004

[6] Chikungunya virus in the United States. 2018. Available from: https://www.cdc.gov/chikungunya/geo/united-states.html [Accessed: 24 February 2019]

[7] Yactayo S et al. Epidemiology of chikungunya in the Americas. The Journal of Infectious Diseases. 2016;**214**(suppl 5):S441-S445

[8] Zeller H, Van Bortel W, Sudre B. Chikungunya: Its history in Africa and Asia and its spread to new regions in 2013-2014. The Journal of Infectious Diseases. 2016;**214**(suppl 5):S436-S440

[9] Charlys da Costa A et al. Spread of chikungunya virus east/central/south African genotype in Northeast Brazil. Emerging Infectious Diseases. 2017;**23**(10):1742-1744

[10] Goupil BA, Mores CN. A review of chikungunya virus-induced arthralgia: Clinical manifestations, therapeutics, and pathogenesis. The Open Rheumatology Journal. 2016;**10**:129-140

[11] Sergon K et al. Seroprevalence of chikungunya virus infection on Grande Comore Island, union of the Comoros, 2005. The American Journal of Tropical Medicine and Hygiene. 2007;**76**(6):1189-1193

[12] Pinheiro TJ et al. Neurological manifestations of chikungunya and zika infections. Arquivos de Neuro-Psiquiatria. 2016;**74**(11):937-943

[13] Mahendradas P, Avadhani K, Shetty R. Chikungunya and the eye: A review. Journal of Ophthalmic Inflammation and Infection. 2013;**3**(1):35

[14] Simon F, Paule P, Oliver M. Chikungunya virus-induced myopericarditis: Toward an increase of dilated cardiomyopathy in countries with epidemics? The American Journal of Tropical Medicine and Hygiene. 2008;**78**(2):212-213

[15] Alvarez MF et al. Cardiovascular involvement and manifestations of systemic chikungunya virus infection: A systematic review. F1000Research. 2017;**6**:390

[16] Simon F et al. French guidelines for the management of chikungunya (acute and persistent presentations). November 2014. Médecine et Maladies Infectieuses. 2015;**45**(7):243-263

[17] Cardona-Ospina JA et al. Mortality and fatality due to chikungunya virus infection in Colombia. Journal of Clinical Virology. 2015;**70**:14-15

[18] Freitas ARR et al. Excess mortality related to chikungunya epidemics in the context of co-circulation of

other arboviruses in Brazil. PLoS Currents. 2017;**9**:ecurrents.outbreaks.14608e586cd321d8d5088652d7a0d884

[19] Economopoulou A et al. Atypical chikungunya virus infections: Clinical manifestations, mortality and risk factors for severe disease during the 2005-2006 outbreak on Reunion. Epidemiology and Infection. 2009;**137**(4):534-541

[20] Schuffenecker I et al. Genome microevolution of chikungunya viruses causing the Indian Ocean outbreak. PLoS Medicine. 2006;**3**(7):e263

[21] Schilte C et al. Chikungunya virus-associated long-term arthralgia: A 36-month prospective longitudinal study. PLoS Neglected Tropical Diseases. 2013;**7**(3):e2137

[22] Rodriguez-Morales AJ et al. Post-chikungunya chronic inflammatory rheumatism: Results from a retrospective follow-up study of 283 adult and child cases in La Virginia, Risaralda, Colombia. F1000Research. 2016;**5**:360

[23] Mathew AJ et al. Rheumatic-musculoskeletal pain and disorders in a naive group of individuals 15 months following a chikungunya viral epidemic in South India: A population based observational study. International Journal of Clinical Practice. 2011;**65**(12):1306-1312

[24] Amaral JK, Bingham CO 3rd, Schoen RT. Successful methotrexate treatment of chronic chikungunya arthritis. Journal of Clinical Rheumatology. 2018. DOI: 10.1097/RHU.0000000000000943

[25] Sepulveda-Delgado J et al. Inflammatory biomarkers, disease activity index, and self-reported disability may be predictors of chronic arthritis after chikungunya infection: Brief report. Clinical Rheumatology. 2017;**36**(3):695-699

[26] Zaid A et al. Chikungunya arthritis: Implications of acute and chronic inflammation mechanisms on disease management. Arthritis & Rhematology. 2018;**70**(4):484-495

[27] Ng KW et al. Clinical features and epidemiology of chikungunya infection in Singapore. Singapore Medical Journal. 2009;**50**(8):785-790

[28] Chow A et al. Persistent arthralgia induced by chikungunya virus infection is associated with interleukin-6 and granulocyte macrophage colony-stimulating factor. The Journal of Infectious Diseases. 2011;**203**(2):149-157

[29] Miossec P, Korn T, Kuchroo VK. Interleukin-17 and type 17 helper T cells. The New England Journal of Medicine. 2009;**361**(9):888-898

[30] Chen W et al. Arthritogenic alphaviral infection perturbs osteoblast function and triggers pathologic bone loss. Proceedings of the National Academy of Sciences of the United States of America. 2014;**111**(16):6040-6045

[31] Sourisseau M et al. Characterization of reemerging chikungunya virus. PLoS Pathogens. 2007;**3**(6):e89

[32] Hoarau JJ et al. Persistent chronic inflammation and infection by chikungunya arthritogenic alphavirus in spite of a robust host immune response. Journal of Immunology. 2010;**184**(10):5914-5927

[33] Soden M et al. Detection of viral ribonucleic acid and histologic analysis of inflamed synovium in Ross River virus infection. Arthritis and Rheumatism. 2000;**43**(2):365-369

[34] Labadie K et al. Chikungunya disease in nonhuman primates involves long-term viral persistence in macrophages. The Journal of Clinical Investigation. 2010;**120**(3):894-906

[35] Bouquillard E et al. Rheumatic manifestations associated with chikungunya virus infection: A study of 307 patients with 32-month follow-up (RHUMATOCHIK study). Joint, Bone, Spine. 2018;**85**(2):207-210

[36] Chang AY et al. Chikungunya arthritis mechanisms in the Americas: A cross-sectional analysis of chikungunya arthritis patients twenty-two months after infection demonstrating no detectable viral persistence in synovial fluid. Arthritis & Rhematology. 2018;**70**(4):585-593

[37] Reddy V et al. Molecular mimicry between chikungunya virus and host components: A possible mechanism for the arthritic manifestations. PLoS Neglected Tropical Diseases. 2017;**11**(1):e0005238

[38] Manimunda SP et al. Clinical progression of chikungunya fever during acute and chronic arthritic stages and the changes in joint morphology as revealed by imaging. Transactions of the Royal Society of Tropical Medicine and Hygiene. 2010;**104**(6):392-399

[39] Javelle E et al. Specific management of post-chikungunya rheumatic disorders: A retrospective study of 159 cases in Reunion Island from 2006-2012. PLoS Neglected Tropical Diseases. 2015;**9**(3):e0003603

[40] Simon F et al. Chikungunya infection: An emerging rheumatism among travelers returned from Indian Ocean islands. Report of 47 cases. Medicine (Baltimore). 2007;**86**(3):123-137

[41] Sissoko D et al. Post-epidemic chikungunya disease on Reunion Island: Course of rheumatic manifestations and associated factors over a 15-month period. PLoS Neglected Tropical Diseases. 2009;**3**(3):e389

[42] Padmakumar B et al. Comparative evaluation of four therapeutic regimes in chikungunya arthritis: A prospective randomized parallel-group study. Indian Journal of Rheumatology. 2009;**4**(3):94-101

[43] Brighton SW. Chloroquine phosphate treatment of chronic chikungunya arthritis. An open pilot study. South African Medical Journal. 1984;**66**(6):217-218

[44] Brito CA et al. Pharmacologic management of pain in patients with chikungunya: A guideline. Revista da Sociedade Brasileira de Medicina Tropical. 2016;**49**(6):668-679

[45] De Lamballerie X et al. On chikungunya acute infection and chloroquine treatment. Vector Borne and Zoonotic Diseases. 2008;**8**(6):837-839

[46] Chopra A, Saluja M, Venugopalan A. Effectiveness of chloroquine and inflammatory cytokine response in patients with early persistent musculoskeletal pain and arthritis following chikungunya virus infection. Arthritis & Rhematology. 2014;**66**(2):319-326

[47] Ravindran V, Alias G. Efficacy of combination DMARD therapy vs. hydroxychloroquine monotherapy in chronic persistent chikungunya arthritis: A 24-week randomized controlled open label study. Clinical Rheumatology. 2017;**36**(6):1335-1340

[48] Ganu MA, Ganu AS. Post-chikungunya chronic arthritis—Our experience with DMARDs over two year follow up. The Journal of the Association of Physicians of India. 2011;**59**:83-86

[49] Pandya s. Methotrexate and hydroxychloroquine combination therapy in chronic chikungunya

arthritis: A 16 week study. Indian Journal of Rheumatology. 2008;**3**(3):93-97

[50] Bouquillard E, Combe B. A report of 21 cases of rheumatoid arthritis following chikungunya fever. A mean follow-up of two years. Joint, Bone, Spine. 2009;**76**(6):654-657

[51] Zaid A et al. Disease exacerbation by etanercept in a mouse model of alphaviral arthritis and myositis. Arthritis and Rheumatism. 2011;**63**(2):488-491

[52] Miner JJ et al. Therapy with CTLA4-Ig and an antiviral monoclonal antibody controls chikungunya virus arthritis. Science Translational Medicine. 2017;**9**(375):eaah3438

[53] Herrero LJ et al. Pentosan polysulfate: A novel glycosaminoglycan-like molecule for effective treatment of alphavirus-induced cartilage destruction and inflammatory disease. Journal of Virology. 2015;**89**(15):8063-8076

[54] Teo TH et al. Fingolimod treatment abrogates chikungunya virus-induced arthralgia. Science Translational Medicine. 2017;**9**(375):eaal1333

Section 2

Zoonotic Diseases

Chapter 5

More than a Hundred Years in the Search for an Accurate Diagnosis for Chagas Disease: Current Panorama and Expectations

Aracely López-Monteon, Eric Dumonteil and Angel Ramos-Ligonio

Abstract

Chagas disease, or American trypanosomiasis, is a parasitic disease of the Americas. In nature, *Trypanosoma cruzi* is transmitted through various species of triatomine bugs. However, non-vectorial transmission can also occur, such as transmission through blood products or by transplanting infected organs, by vertical transmission, and lately by oral route. Currently, Chagas disease affects approximately 6–7 million people worldwide, and the process of urbanization in Latin America and migratory movements from endemic countries have led to Chagas disease being diagnosed in areas where the infection is not endemic. There are several methods for diagnosing Chagas disease. Some of these are mostly used for research purposes, while others are used in routine diagnostic laboratories. According to the World Health Organization (WHO), chronic Chagas disease diagnosis is based on two serological techniques. To establish a definitive diagnosis, the results must be concordant. In the case of discordances, the WHO proposes repeating serology in a new sample, and if results remain inconclusive, a confirmatory test should be performed. This chapter shows aspects of the diagnosis of Chagas disease, which varies in its sensitivity and specificity, and its use depends on the geographical location, the available resources, and the purpose of the diagnosis.

Keywords: chagas disease, *T. cruzi*, diagnosis, serology, antigens

1. Introduction

The infection caused by the protozoan parasite *Trypanosoma cruzi* leads to Chagas disease, with an estimated 6–7 million infected people and nearly 60 million at risk of infection [1, 2]. Chagas disease ranks among the world's most neglected diseases and is considered to be the parasitic infection with the greatest socioeconomic impact in Latin America, being responsible for an estimated US$ 1.2 billion in lost productivity annually [3]. It is a disease that a century after its discovery still requires appropriate control measures, effective treatment, and especially an accurate diagnosis. This disease is endemic to most countries in Latin America [4], but it has now become more important in other regions. The increasing presence of Chagas in non-endemic areas, as well as the resurgence of the disease in endemic countries, has been a major focus of attention in recent years [5] and, over the last 40 years, has become a global health concern due to the huge migration flows from Latin America to Europe, United States, Canada, and Japan. In Europe, most migrants from Chagas disease-endemic areas are concentrated in Spain, Italy, France, United Kingdom, and Switzerland (**Figure 1**) [6]. The flagellate protozoa *T. cruzi* is usually transmitted through infected feces and/or urine excreted by triatomines (Hemiptera: Reduviidae) during blood feeding. However, this is a nonlinear phenomenon, as mammals can be exposed to infection multiple times through distinct routes [7]; the main routes of transmission of the parasite are through the insect vector, blood transfusion, transplants of organs, congenital via, orally and it is now reported that the infection is capable of being transmitted sexually (**Figure 2**). In addition, the fact that Chagas disease can be transmitted sexually, along with the migration problems of individuals affected with Chagas disease to countries that were previously not endemic, and travel to endemic countries, has direct implications for public health for the spread of this disease [8], the transmission through vector only occurs in endemic areas for this disease. In non-endemic countries, the main routes of transmission are blood and congenital transmission [9–11]. *T. cruzi* has a high genetic diversity, which is why it has been classified into discrete typing units (DTU): TCI-TcVI, in addition, of a genotype associated with bats (TcBat); this classification was made based on different characteristics such as geographical distribution and clinical manifestations of the disease, among others. As TcI is the most widely distributed DTU and with a wide genetic diversity, it has been divided into domestic and sylvatic genotypes (TcIDom and TcISyl) [12].

The disease presents two phases. In the acute phase, ranging from the time of infection until about 6 weeks after this, patients present a high parasitemia and may show nonspecific symptoms, such as fever and headache. During the chronic phase, which can last up to 30 years, approximately 30% of patients develop cardiac complications such as arrhythmias and cardiomyopathy, and 10% of patients may present intestinal complications, especially constipation, or neurological complications. However, the chronic phase is characterized by the absence of symptoms in most patients (**Figure 3**) [1, 13]. The latter, coupled with the fact that patients can be found in non-endemic areas where the disease is unknown, represents an added difficulty for the diagnosis of infection [14]. The effectiveness of methods for diagnosing infectious diseases depends on their sensitivity and specificity for the unambiguous detection of the presence of the pathogen or the specific host

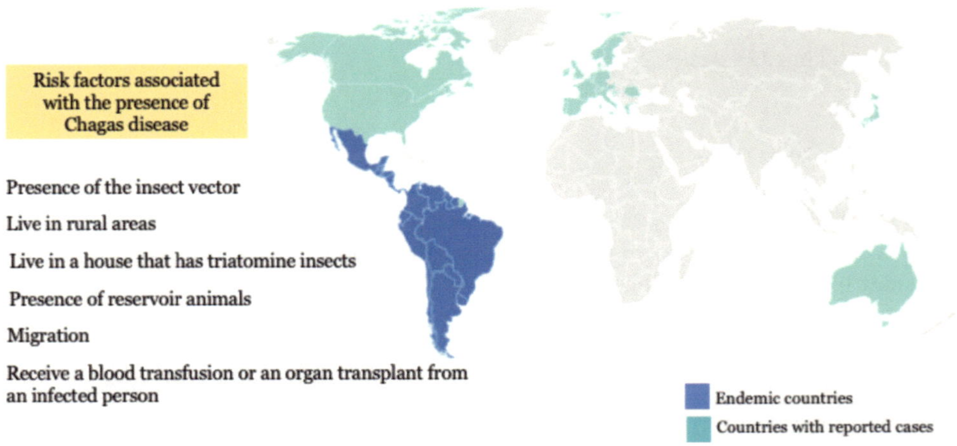

Figure 1.
Distribution of Chagas Disease (WHO: Estimated data 2010).

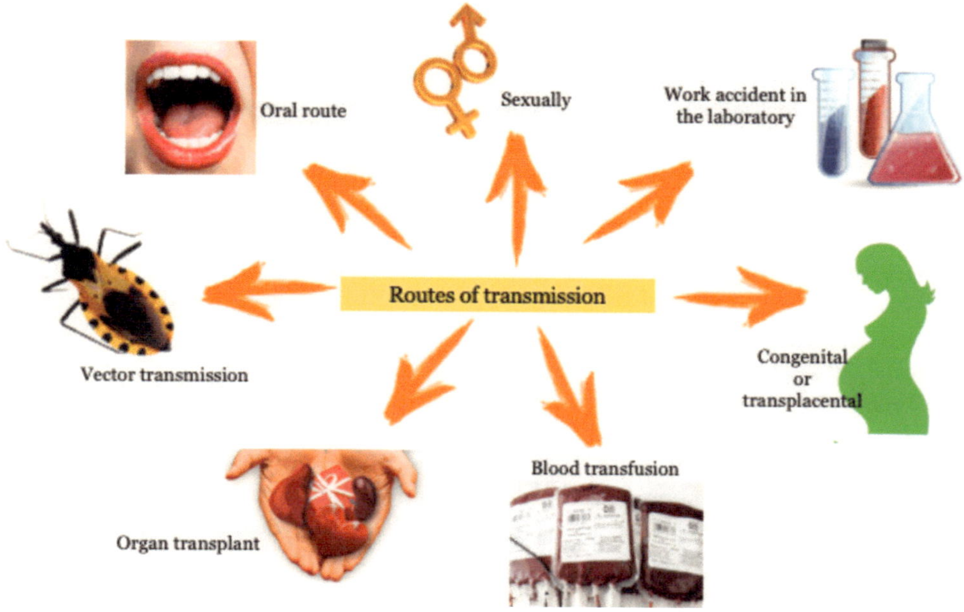

Figure 2.
Main routes of transmission of the Trypanosoma cruzi.

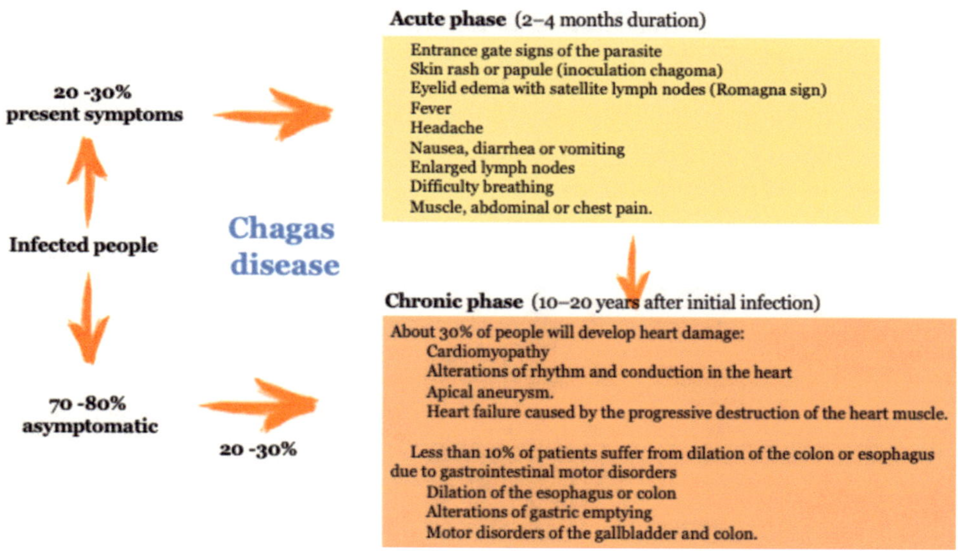

Figure 3.
Chagas disease has two stages or clinical phases: an acute phase and a chronic phase. People (from 70 to 80% of those infected) are asymptomatic throughout their lives, but from 20 to 30% of those affected, this disease progresses to chronic symptoms.

response in response to infection. New technologies based on molecular biology have enabled the identification of biomarkers exclusive of infectious agents, molecules involved in interactions with their hosts, and of the host molecules which mediate response to infection [15]. Infectious diseases remain a major public health problem worldwide. In this scenario, the immunodiagnostic method has been and will remain an essential tool to demonstrate the presence of infection in patients, for disease prognosis, for monitoring clinical studies, and, also, as tools to monitor the success of strategies for control and epidemiological monitoring [16]. Finally, this chapter was conceived to the current need for an accurate diagnosis for Chagas disease, since the correct diagnosis is a priority not only to identify the people who should receive the appropriate treatment but also to reduce and prevent the risk of transmission through a blood transfusion or an organ transplant.

2. Why the need for an accurate diagnosis for Chagas disease

One of the limitations for the prevention and control of neglected tropical diseases is that the sociocultural aspects associated with diseases are ignored. Cases of Chagas disease in endemic areas occur in specific contexts marked by sociocultural, political, and economic circumstances. In addition, in the case of Chagas disease, the absence of symptoms in most cases, the lack of ability to detect and/or identify the disease, the lack of information on services and immigration policies, affect. It is very important to be able to obtain prevention and control measures for the disease, even in non-endemic countries [17]. Understanding this behavior can allow to guide health policies to combat these types of diseases, where indigenous groups and children are considered especially vulnerable groups.

2.1 The current status of the diagnosis of Chagas disease

Diagnostic methods for *T. cruzi* can be included in three main groups: parasitological, serological, and molecular (**Figure 4**). Parasitological methods aim to visualize the presence of parasites, and their sensitivity varies depending on the stage of infection [18]. For diagnosis of the disease in the phase where the parasitemia is very low, immunological methods (serological) are based primarily on the search for G antibodies (IgG) anti-*T. cruzi* in the blood of patients and their colorimetric reaction visible in the case that the blood of the patients contains the antibodies. [19]. The most commonly used methods are ELISA test (sensitivity = 94–100%, specificity = 96–100%), indirect hemagglutination (HAI, sensitivity = 88–99%, specificity = 96–100%), and indirect immunofluorescence (IFI, sensitivity = 98%, specificity = 98%). Despite being highly sensitive and specific, serological tests can have some cross-reactivity.

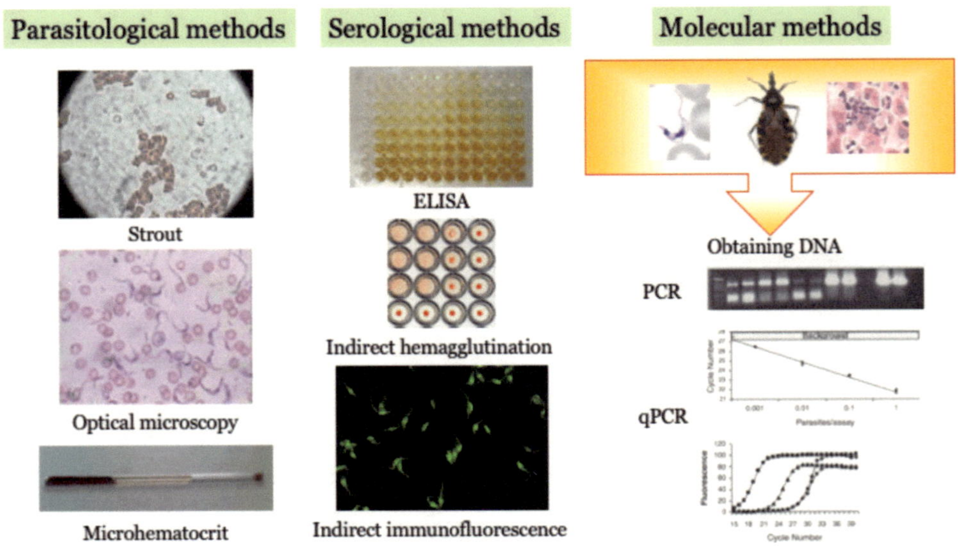

Figure 4.
Diagnostic methods for T. cruzi.

Another technique based on the search for anti-*T. cruzi* antibodies is the Western blot, which has been used in the diagnosis of Chagas disease using mainly excretion-secretion antigens and in some cases recombinant proteins. In the reported works, the Western blot has been used mainly to confirm the serological results obtained when other serological techniques are discordant or when there are cases of cross-reaction with *Leishmania*, and it has been observed that the technique possesses a high sensitivity and specificity. Although this test is not used routinely, and it is not considered as a substitute for conventional serological tests, it may be useful as an additional diagnostic test or for field studies [20–22]. Detection of parasite DNA using molecular diagnostic tools could be an alternative or complement to current diagnostic methods, but its implementation in endemic regions remains limited, due to lack of standardization, complexity, lack of clinical evidence, and the cost of implementation [23].

The application of molecular biological techniques has allowed the production of specific antigens in large quantities for use in immunologic techniques, including recombinant antigens and synthetic peptides [24]. Molecular biology methods are characterized by a high specificity and sensitivity, particularly during the acute phase, and hybridization techniques have been used for the detection of specific DNA fragments of the parasite genome by polymerase chain reaction (PCR) [25–27]. One of the major limitations of the PCR technique in the diagnosis of Chagas disease is its low sensitivity in the chronic phase due to the very low level of circulating parasites, since these are confined to tissues [28, 29]. However, it is important to note that the sensitivity of PCR is also influenced by the method of DNA extraction and the volume of blood that is used for DNA extraction [30]. Parasite detection from organ biopsies is indeed more successful during chronic infection when parasites sequester within organs; however, this technique is impractical because biopsies are not easily collected [31, 32]. Some authors proposed that circulating parasite antigens could be used as highly specific biomarkers of infection by *T. cruzi* as observed in mouse models [33]. Serum proteins have also been proposed as markers of Chagasic patients [34]. However, diagnosis remains mostly focused on the identification of antibodies against the parasite (**Table 1**) [35]. The nature of the antigens used in anti-*T. cruzi* assays is critical for the specificity of the assay, particularly in the case of individuals infected with related protozoan parasites such as *Leishmania*, as epitopes may cross-react with crude *T. cruzi* antigens [36]. Various types of serologic tests are currently used to establish the diagnosis of Chagas disease (**Table 2**), based on total parasite extracts and/or recombinant antigens [37, 38]. These serological assays for detecting antibodies to *T. cruzi* are generally classified as screening or confirmatory assays (**Table 2**). First-line screening assays provide the presumptive identification of antibody-reactive specimens, and supplemental assays are used to confirm whether samples found reactive with a particular screening assay do indeed contain antibodies specific to *T. cruzi*. When a single screening assay is used for testing in a population with a very low prevalence of Chagas disease, the probability that an individual is infected when a reactive test result is obtained (i.e., the positive predictive value) is very low, since the majority of individuals with reactive results are not infected. This problem occurs even when an assay with high specificity is used. Accuracy can be improved if a second supplemental assay is used to retest all those specimens found reactive by the first assay. Those found non-reactive by the assay are considered negative for antibodies to *T. cruzi*. Serum/plasma samples with low antibody titer are frequently found in individuals from endemic regions. In general, those samples are difficult to confirm and give a definitive final status. The clinical significance of these samples and associated potential risk of transmission by an individual presenting with low antibody titer is also little understood. These could represent individuals spontaneous cure or treated by current

Diagnostic methods in the acute phase
Direct methods without concentration
Direct methods of concentration
• Microhematocrit • Strout test
Diagnostic methods in the chronic phase
Serology • ELISA • Indirect immunofluorescence • Indirect hemagglutination
Other parasitological and molecular biology methods* • Xenodiagnostic • In vitro culture • PCR

**Can be used in any phase, with low parasitemia, and is not detected by other methods.*

Table 1.
Diagnoses for chagas disease.

antiparasitic medication [39] or have cross-reactivity with other agents such as *Leishmania* [40]. To date, and according to the WHO, an individual is diagnosed as infected with *T. cruzi* in the chronic phase of the disease when the results of two serological tests are positive, due to the different immunogenicity of different strains of the parasite, different immune responses between patients, and the existence of cross-reactions with other trypanosomatids coexisting in endemic areas when using crude parasite antigens [16, 38]. When inconclusive or discordant results appear, a third technique [38] or additional samples are required [41]. However, during the diagnosis of the disease, we must take into account certain conditions and/or variables that are not directly dependent on the design and development of the test; as in the case of the host response, this depends partly on the strain of parasite and secondly on the genetic background of the host [42]. Moreover, the existence of the "immunological memory" in models where there was a parasitological cure suggests that parasite antigens may persist in some organs, which could be inducing the production of antibodies, regardless of the presence of live parasite [43, 44]. In patients treated during the chronic phase, the objective is to analyze a tendency for negativization of the serological tests, which requires to monitor patients for many years following treatment. This has brought controversies regarding the criterion of a serologic cure [45, 46]. Some researchers believe that a reduction in antibody titers after a prolonged time can be considered as a criterion of cure, in contrast to others who recommend total negativization of serological tests [47]. In areas where Chagas disease is endemic, the choice among ELISA, IIF, or IHA for serological testing is based on availability [31, 32, 38, 48]. However, these techniques may be unspecific as they can cross-react with other parasites [49]. Because of this cross-reaction, the use of antigen secretion/excretion of parasite in diagnostic tests has been proposed. It has been shown that proteins from trypomastigotes are better antigens to detect antibodies against the parasite; however, most antigens used for immunological tests are total protein extracts derived from epimastigotes, because of the ease of

DOI: http://dx.doi.org/10.5772/intechopen.86567

Test	Antigen	Manufacturer	Country
Immunoenzymatic assay			
AccuDiag™ Chagas ELISA Kit	NI	Diagnostic Automation/ Cortez Diagnostics, Inc.	USA
ImmunoComb® II Chagas Ab Kit	RA	Alere Inc.	Germany
Anti-Chagas IgG ELISA Kit	NI	Abcam	United Kingdom
Abbott ESA Chagas	Purified antigens	Abbott Laboratories	USA
Abbott PRISM Chagas	Purified antigens	Abbott Laboratories	USA
T. cruzi Ab (Chagas)		Bioars	Argentina
EIAgen *Trypanosoma cruzi* Ab	Total extract	Adaltis	Italy
Chagas screen ELISA	Cytoplasmic membrane antigen	Wiener lab	Argentina
Chagas ELISA IgG + IgM	RA	Vircell	Spain
Pathozyme Chagas	RA	Omega Diagnostics Limited	Scotland
Chagas Rec ELISA	RA	Human Diagnostics Worldwide	Germany
Chagas ELISA	Total extract	Ebram Produtos Laboratoriais Ltda	Brazil
Chagatek ELISA	Purified antigens	Laboratório Lemos SRL	Argentina
NovaLisa Chagas (*Trypanosoma cruzi*)	NI	NovaTec Immundiagnostica	Germany
Premier Chagas IgG ELISA test	Purified antigens	Meridian Diagnostics	USA
Test ELISA para Chagas	Total extract strain (Tulahuén and Mn)	BIOSChile	Chile
Bio-Manguinhos EIA	Total extract/RP	Bio-Manguinhos	Brazil
IVD ELISA	NI	IVD Research Inc.	USA
DRG®*Trypanosoma cruzi* IgG	NI	DRG International Inc.	USA
Chagas IgG ELISA	RA	Gull Laboratories Inc./ Meridian Bioscience Inc.	USA
Cellabs *T. cruzi* IgG CELISA	NI	Cellabs Pty Ltd.	Australia
BIOELISACRUZI	Total extract	Biolab-Mérieux	Brazil
Dia Kit Bio-Chagas	RA	Gador SA	Argentina
BIOZIMA Chagas kit	Purified antigens	Laboratório Lemos SRL	Argentina
Abbott Chagas Anticorpos EIA	RA	Abbott Laboratories	USA
Cruzi TEST ELISA	NI	GenCell Biosystems	Ireland
Chagas test *IICS*, ELISA	Total extract (Y strain)	IICS Univ de Asunción	Paraguay
HBK 401 Hemobio Chagas	Total extract	Embrabio	Brazil
Chagatest ELISA	Total extract/RP	Wiener lab	Argentina
Bioelisa Chagas	Synthetic peptides	Biokit	Spain
Chagas Hemagen	Purified antigens	Hemagen Diagnósticos	USA

Test	Antigen	Manufacturer	Country
BioMérieux	Total extract/RP	BioMérieux	France
BLK	Total extract	BLK diagnostics	Spain
Siemens IMMULITE Chagas IgG	RA	Siemens Healthcare	USA
Anti-Chagas Symbiosis	NI	Symbiosys	Brazil
ORTHO *T. cruzi* ELISA Test System	Total extract	Jhonson and Jhonson	USA
Certest	(Strain Tulahuen and Mn)	Abbott Laboratories	Spain
ImmunoComb II Chagas Ab	RA/peptides	Orgenics	Israel
Elecsys Chagas assay	Recombinant antigens	Roche Diagnostic	
Gold ELISA Chagas	Recombinant proteins and purified lysates		Brazil
ELISA Chagas III	Total extract	Grupo Bios	Chile
Imuno-ELISA Chagas	Recombinant antigens	Wama Diagnóstica	Brazil
T. cruzi Ab, DIAPRO	Recombinant antigens	Diagnostic BioProbes	Italy
Trypanosoma cruzi IgG ELISA Kit	Total extract	MyBiosource	USA
Chagas (*Trypanosoma cruzi*) IgG assay	NI	DEMEDITEC Diagnostics GmbH	Germany
Chagas (*Trypanosoma cruzi*) IgG ELISA	NI	GenWay Biotech, Inc.	USA
Chagas (*Trypanosoma cruzi*) IgG ELISA	NI	IBL International GmbH	Germany
CELQUEST CHAGAS ELISA	Recombinant antigens	ATGen Diagnostica	Italy
Immunochromatographic assay			
OnSite Chagas Ab Rapid test	RA	CTK Biotech	USA
Chagas AB Rapid	RA	Standard Diagnostics	Korea
WL Check Chagas	RA	Wiener Lab	Argentina
Chagas Instantest	Antigens attached to colloidal gold	Silanes	Mexico
Prueba rápida Chagas	Antigens attached to colloidal gold	Amunet Labarotarios	Mexico
Chagas Detect™ Plus	Multi-epitope recombinant antigen	InBios, Inc.	USA
Chagas-certum	Antigens attached to colloidal gold	Certum® Diagnostics	Mexico
Chagas Quick Test	Multi-epitope recombinant antigen	Cypress Diagnostic	Belgium
Chagas Stat-Pak assay	RA	Chembio Diagnostic Systems	USA
PATH-Lemos rapid test	RA	Laboratório Lemos SRL	Argentina
Immu-Sure Chagas (*T. cruzi*)		Millennium Biotech	USA

Test	Antigen	Manufacturer	Country
SD Chagas Ab Rapid	RA	Standard Diagnostic	Korea
ICT Operon	Purified antigens	Operon	Spain
Hemagglutination assays			
Chagas HAI Imunoserum	Sheep red blood cells are sensitized by binding *T. cruzi* antigen	Laboratório Lemos SRL	Argentina
ID-PaGIA, version 2 Ag/version 3 Ag	RA/purified antigens	DiaMed	Switzerland
Chagatest IHA	Erythrocytes sensitized with parasite lysate	Wiener	Argentina
Chagas HAI	Bird red blood cells are sensitized by binding purified *T. cruzi* (Y strain)	Ebram	Brazil
Imuno-HAI Chagas	Bird red blood cells are sensitized by binding purified *T. cruzi* (Y strain)	WAMA	Brazil
Chagas Hemagen HA	Human red blood cells are sensitized by binding epimastigote and amastigote forms of *T. cruzi* (Y and CL strain)	Hemagen Diagnosticos	USA
Hemacruzi	Erythrocytes sensitized with parasite lysate	Biolab-Mérieux	Brazil
ID-Chagas antibody test	Gel particles coated with peptides	DiaMed-ID	Switzerland
Serodia Chagas	Gelatin particles coated with inactivated *Trypanosoma cruzi* antigens	Fujirebio, Inc.	Japan
Immunofluorescence assays			
Chagas IFA	NI	Vircell	Spain
Inmunofluor Chagas kit	Epimastigotes	Biocientífica S.A	Argentina
Kit Trypanosomiasis IFI	Epimastigotes	Tryniti-Mardx (Inverness Medical)	USA
Inmunofluor Chagas IFI	Parasites NI	Biocientífica S.A. (Inverness Medical)	Argentina
MarDx IFA		MarDx Diagnostics, Inc.	USA
IFA Kit Trypanosomiasis		Innogenetics Ibérica	Spain

Test	Antigen	Manufacturer	Country
Chemiluminescent immunoassay			
Architect Chagas assay (prototype) immunoparticles	RA	Abbott Laboratories	Spain
CHAGAS VIRCLIA	NI	Vircell	Spain
PCR assays			
T. cruzi OligoC-TesT	NA	Coris BioConcept	Belgium
AMPLIRUN® TRYPANOSOMA DNA CONTROL	NA	Vircell	Spain
Loop-mediated isothermal amplification (LAMP) assay	NA	Eiken Chemical Company	China
RealCycler CHAG	NA	Progenie Molecular	Spain
TCRUZIDNA.CE	NA	Diagnostic Bioprobes Srl	Italy
RealStar® Chagas PCR Kit RUO	NA	altona Diagnostics GmbH	Germany
VIASURE *Trypanosoma cruzi* Real Time PCR Detection Kit	NA	Certets Biotec	Spain
Confirmatory assays			
Radioimmunoprecipitation analysis [RIPA]	Radiolabeled *T. cruzi* surface antigens	University of Iowa	USA
INNO-LIA Chagas assay	Recombinant and synthetic *T. cruzi* antigens	Innogenetics	Belgium
IF Imunocruzi	Epimastigotes	Biolab Mérieux	Brazil
TESA-blot	Excreted-secreted antigens	Biolab Mérieux	Brazil
Multiplex Immunoassay Multi-cruzi (prototype)	Protein array	NA	NA

RA, recombinant antigen; NI, not indicated; NA, not applicable.

Table 2.
List of commercial diagnostic tests for the serological detection of T. cruzi (Chagas disease).

obtaining them, at lower cost and the presence of common antigens with trypomastigotes [50]. Nevertheless, these tests also show cases of false negatives and cross-reactivity [51–56]. Due to the complexity of the interaction of *T. cruzi* with its host, a single recombinant antigen has not reached the efficacy shown by the total extracts of the parasite. Thus, the antigenic composition of the tests based on recombinant antigens includes a combination of several epitopes [57]. Flow cytometry has mainly been used for differential diagnosis between Chagas disease and leishmaniasis owing to cross-reactivity. Even with optimized serological assays that use parasite-specific recombinant antigens, inconclusive test results continue to be a problem [58]. However, this technique is utilized for monitoring treatments rather than for diagnosis [59]. In the past decade, several technologies have emerged as diagnostic tools capable of improving diagnosis by using several antigens. The diagnostic process becomes faster and less expensive, and the hands-on time in laboratories decreases substantially since these platforms can be fully automated. A multiplex assay platform was evaluated to detect *T. cruzi* infection using the recombinant antigens CRA, FRA, CRA-FRA fusion and parasite lysate; these antigens presented different sensitivity and specificity by themselves; however, when mixed they increased its sensitivity and specificity, suggesting that they could be an alternative to single-test detection for Chagas disease [60]. Moreover, the immunochromatography represents a promising method which can be performed with whole blood, and it has many advantages over most existing diagnostic methods, requires little time, and does not require trained personnel; its main advantage is that it can be used in field work [61], but there are cases of discordance [62]. However, despite that, there are reports where it manifests that it no longer needed investing so much in research and development for the diagnosis of Chagas disease, because that rapid tests on the market are sufficiently valid both in America and in Europe and Asia-Pacific [63]; however, this is not entirely true, since several studies have shown discordance between the various commercial techniques. As mentioned, the diagnosis of Chagas disease is based mainly on serological tests because parasitemia is generally low or cannot be detected during the chronic phase of the infection. Finally, low reaction samples may not be detectable by all serological assays; besides, the presence of the so-called "serosilent" infections [64], in which parasitemia is detectable in seronegative individuals, represents a potential risk to acquire the parasite.

2.2 The world of diagnosis for Chagas disease: a discordant paradise

The accurate diagnosis of *T. cruzi* infection is pivotal to the clinical management of Chagas disease. *T. cruzi* has a complex life cycle, and its ability to infect any nucleated cell complicates diagnosis [65]. Additionally, the absence of a "gold standard" test that reliably and consistently detects the presence of a *T. cruzi* infection makes the evaluation of current methods difficult [28, 66]. Serodiscordance in Chagas disease remains a challenge since individuals with inconclusive results are clinically complicated to manage [67]; this problem usually arises in the diagnosis during the chronic phase. Performing two or more serological testing does not guarantee that the result shall be univocal. It is called serodiscordance when in the same patient two tests give different results (frequent situation during treatment, in pregnant patients or patient in acute cases), because the main criterion for "cure" has been the conversion to negative serology on all tests performed. However, this result is often not observed until 8–10 years posttreatment and then only in approximately 15% of treated adult subjects [68]. Experts recommend that the IFI which has a sensitivity of 95% and a specificity of 100% is used. However, it is often not the most advisable since reading can be subjective, depending on the experience of the technician. Another situation that often occurs in reading spectrophotometric tests, such as ELISA, is that the values of optical density (OD) are very close to the cutoff value (±10%), in which case the result should not be considered positive or negative but rather indeterminate. Alternatives have been proposed as IFI, antigens' parasite excretion-secretion (TESA) used in ELISA or immunoblot assays or by radioimmunoassay (RIPA), or various recombinant antigens used in immunoblot [14]. To date no test alone can establish the diagnosis or confirmation of infection by *T. cruzi* nor rule out the problem of cross-reactivity; the combination of tests usually generates discrepant results, often in a limited number of cases. Some commercial tests have very limited ability to detect *T. cruzi* infection in populations of particular study; internal tests based on crude parasite antigens showed a higher sensitivity but were still unable to detect all cases of *T. cruzi* infection [69], for example, the University of Sao Paulo conducted tests to detect *T. cruzi* antibodies using the three methods IH, IIF, and ELISA; 4000 serum samples were analyzed, of which only 1901 (48%) were positive for all three tests, 718 (18%) were negative, and 1381 (35%) had a questionable or inconclusive results. The discrepancies were attributable to the type of parasite antigen; IIF detects a specific antibody that reacts with a parasite membrane antigen, whereas HI detects an antibody that reacts with a subcellular antigen. Each of these serological reactions operates in different specificity systems [70]. Another study in Spain was found to have a higher sensitivity (97–100%), and for serological screening of *T. cruzi* infection, a combination of tests is needed [71]. Finally, in a study conducted in a rural community in Veracruz, Mexico, using a combination of five ELISA tests based on different antigenic preparations (two in-house enzyme-linked immunosorbent assay based on crude extract, Chagatest ELISA recombinant v3.0, Chagatek ELISA, and NovaLisa Chagas), a very high level of discordance (32%) was also found among the ELISA tests used, with very poor agreement among them. This showed that the commercial tests had a very limited ability to detect *T. cruzi* infection, and the in-house tests based on crude parasite antigens showed a greater sensitivity but were still unable to detect all cases of *T. cruzi* infection, even when based on a local parasite strain [69].

To date, *T. cruzi* diagnostic present problems of sensitivity, making the diagnosis confusing and often requiring additional testing [40, 70, 71]. In congenital cases, it has been observed that discordance between the samples analyzed also occurs, and discordant results were confirmed by a third diagnostic test [72]. Although numerous assays are available for diagnosing Chagas disease, no single test is considered the reference standard to confirm the diagnosis of infection by the parasite [73–76]. Serology is a useful tool in the diagnosis of Chagas disease, but in certain circumstances, none of the techniques described above serves as a marker of cure or progression of infection. Some authors mention that the Western blot is suitable for confirmation of infection by *T. cruzi*, so it is strongly recommended for confirmation and discrimination of discordant cases [22, 77], because this technique has a sensitivity of 86.6% [20, 78], 99% [79], and 100% [80, 81] and a specificity of 100%, making it more effective than techniques such as ELISA, HAI, and IIF. The adequate choice of *T. cruzi* strains as antigen source for the diagnosis of Chagas disease is still controversial due to differences in terms of accuracy reported between different diagnostic tests. The results of this study showed that the sensitivity index did not vary, with percentages of 100% for all strains in both tests. However, the specificity index for the ELISA tests showed differences between 92 and 98% but was reduced to 78–89% when the *Leishmania*-positive sera were included [82].

2.3 Looking for the correct diagnosis

After more than a century of the discovery of Chagas disease, there is no consensus on the choice of a reference technique. Studies in South America reported a high efficiency of commercial kits manufactured in this region [40, 83]. However, work carried out in Central America shows that the use of antigens prepared from *T. cruzi* strains that are isolated in these areas increases the sensitivity of antibody detection assays [69, 84, 85]. This could be due to the predominance of the lineage TcI in the region [86] and the wide expansion of genotypes TcII–TcVI reported in the Southern Cone countries [87]; but lately, the presence of additional DTUs has been demonstrated in countries such as Mexico and the United States [88, 89]. The development of new diagnostics is partially limited by the availability of well-characterized antigens, in addition to the great variability among strains and DTUs in terms of virulence, infectivity, tissue tropism, progression of disease, drug susceptibility, and geographical distribution [31, 90–92]. However, there is as yet no clear association between genetic variants of the parasite and these life history or epidemiological characteristics. Several recombinant antigens that have serologic utility have been identified. However, the most effective antigens have been those with immunodominant, repeating B-cell epitopes [93]. The use of recombinant antigens and/or synthetic peptides has been proposed [94] to improve specificity and sensitivity, which is essential if false-positive or false-negative results are to be avoided. Peptide analysis is a technique widely used for mapping of linear epitopes in proteins from pathogens [95, 96].

The recent availability of peptide microarrays allows rapid and inexpensive serological diagnosis with high performance [97, 98]. The availability of complete pathogen genomes has renewed interest in the development of diagnostics for infectious diseases. Synthetic peptide microarrays provide a rapid, high-throughput platform for immunological testing of potential B-cell epitopes. Therefore, computational approaches for prediction and/or prioritization of diagnostically relevant peptides are required [99]. Currently, high-density peptide chips for the discovery of linear B-cell epitopes' specific pathogens from clinical samples provide the basis for the detection of biomarkers and proteome-scale studies of the immune response against pathogens [100].

The challenge for this process is to identify, by bioinformatics within a given proteome, peptides that could be good targets for a B-cell response. A number of algorithms have been developed for computational prediction of B-cell epitopes [101]. Computational prediction of B-cell epitopes is still an active research field, and a number of state-of-the-art predictors show improved performance [102–105]. As a consequence, predicting diagnostic epitopes in the context of a particular disease or infection is a complex problem, where many additional limitations are not taken into account, such as the mechanism of invasion of infectious agents, the expression pattern of parasite proteins. All these additional variables affect the outcome of the immune response and may explain the observed variability in responses [99]. In recent years, microarray technology has been of great interest, offering valuable opportunities to study the function of genes and the development of diagnostics. The main advantage of a microarray assay is to determine different analytes simultaneously, and it is more sensitive and faster than the conventional ELISA system. Peptide microarrays combined with a bioinformatics peptide selection strategy constitute a powerful and cost-effective platform for serodiagnostic biomarker screening of infectious diseases just as Chagas disease [100]. The development of efficient methods for the detection of microspots with high sensitivity and specificity will enable new applications in future studies applied to protein microarrays [106, 107].

New-generation tests with potentially improved accuracy have been developed recently. The use of a large mixture of recombinant antigens and the incorporation of different detection systems, such as chemiluminescence, increase the sensitivity and specificity of the techniques. Other advantages of new-generation tests are automation, rapidity, and high performance, such as the Architect Chagas or Bio-Flash Chagas (Biokit, Lliçà d'Amunt, Spain), which have improved the diagnosis of Chagas disease with innovative new tools (large mixture of recombinant antigens and chemiluminescence as detection system). Previous studies have also proposed a chemiluminescent ELISA (CL-ELISA) with purified trypomastigote glycoproteins for the detection of lytic protective antibodies against *T. cruzi* in human serum [35, 108–110]. Detection systems, such as chemiluminescence, increase light amplification and signal duration in comparison with traditional ELISAs, which may be a point in favor of these new methodologies, leading to higher accuracy in the diagnosis of Chagas disease. Further studies with other new-generation techniques with similar characteristics (recombinant antigens and chemiluminescence) are necessary [35]. The use of a single technique would reduce diagnosis costs and therefore allow the application of screening and control programs in countries where such systems have not yet been implemented. Previous studies on the cost-effectiveness of Chagas disease management have been undertaken, but the costs of different diagnostic methods have not been compared [111–114]. Thus, several groups have implemented the usage of PCR to the identification of the genetic material from the parasite, in blood and serum samples as well as tissue samples. Several types of the PCR techniques are available to detect *T. cruzi* DNA in serum and blood samples; among them we find conventional PCR, hot-start PCR, and nested PCR. Several tools that use probes to verify the presence/absence of specific DNA are also used; such as: Southern Blot or PCR and hybridization and real-time PCR. An important advantage that the use of PCR offers as a diagnosis tool is that it allows the characterization of the circulating strains in an endemic area for Chagas disease [115]. Finally, there is a need to develop new non-serological non-PCR-based assays to address the limitations of the current methods available for *T. cruzi* detection. For this purpose, assays that detect biomarkers of Chagas disease need to be developed. Biomarker discovery studies reported for Chagas disease lead to the identification of characteristics of host origin, such as host proteins or immune markers, which were elevated in Chagas disease [116, 117]. However, one cannot exclude the possibility that these host markers could also be modulated in conditions unrelated to *T. cruzi* infection, and thus these biomarkers have limited specificity [118]. In order to overcome the issues of specificity, the detection of pathogen-specific factors would be ideal biomarkers of *T. cruzi* infection [33].

3. Conclusions

Chagas disease causes 12,000 deaths each year, and it is estimated that between 7 and 8 million people suffer. This is one of the major public health problems in Latin America. In recent decades, cases have also been detected in North America, Europe, and Asia-Pacific, mainly as a result of migration. An ideal serological test should be easy to perform in a single step, be fast, and be cheap, require no special equipment or refrigeration of reagents, and have 100% sensitivity and specificity; unfortunately, no such test exists for Chagas disease. The lack of a reference standard serological assay for the diagnosis of *T. cruzi* infection has prompted the development of new tests, which require further evaluation, so that the development of diagnostic methods for detecting *T. cruzi* infections, after more than a hundred years of its discovery, remains a challenge which depends mainly on the availability of specific high-affinity antigens. The diagnosis of Chagas disease has limitations, mainly due to the great complexity of the factors that involve it, as well as to the low sensitivity of the parasitological techniques and the low specificity of the immunological tests. Finally, the application of immunomics, which combines serology with proteomics, would help to discover genes and molecules related to the susceptibility and immunity of *T. cruzi* infection, allowing the creation of an adequate diagnosis for the disease, elucidating new therapeutic targets, and, why not, allowing the creation of a vaccine against Chagas disease.

Acknowledgements

This work was supported by grant CONACyT-DCPN-247505-2014.

Conflict of interest

The authors declare no conflict of interest.

Author details

Aracely López-Monteon[1], Eric Dumonteil[2] and Angel Ramos-Ligonio[1]*

1 LADISER Immunology and Molecular Biology, Faculty of Chemistry Science, University of Veracruz, Orizaba, Veracruz, Mexico

2 Department of Tropical Medicine, School of Public Health and Tropical Medicine, Tulane University, New Orleans, LA, USA

*Address all correspondence to: angramos@uv.mx

References

[1] WHO. Chagas Disease (American trypanosomiasis) [Internet]. WHO; 2016. Available from: http://www.who.int/entity/mediacentre/factsheets/fs340/en/index.html

[2] WHO. Reporte del grupo de trabajo científico sobre la enfermedad de Chagas. Geneva: 2017. Available from: http://whqlibdoc.who.int/hq/2007/tDR_SWG_09_spa.pdf

[3] WHO—World Health Organization. Research priorities for Chagas disease, human African trypanosomiasis and leishmaniasis. 2012. Available from: apps.who.int/iris/bitstream/10665/77472/1/WHO_TRS_975_eng.pdf

[4] WHO. Tropical Disease Research. Program for Research and Training Tropical Disease (TDR). Fact Sheet Nu340. Geneva: World Health Organization; 2013

[5] Andrade DV, Gollob KJ, Dutra WO. Acute chagas disease: New global challenges for an old neglected disease. PLoS Neglected Tropical Diseases. 2014;**8**(7):e3010. DOI: 10.1371/journal.pntd.0003010

[6] Antinori S, Galimberti L, Bianco R, Grande R, Galli M, Corbellino M. Chagas disease in Europe: A review for the internist in the globalized world. European Journal of Internal Medicine. 2017;**43**:6-15. DOI: 10.1016/j.ejim.2017.05.001

[7] Jansen AM, Xavier SC, Roque AL. The multiple and complex and changeable scenarios of the *Trypanosoma cruzi* transmission cycle in the sylvatic environment. Acta Tropica. 2015;**151**:1-15

[8] Gomes C, Almeida AB, Rosa AC, Araujo PF, Teixeira ARL. American trypanosomiasis and Chagas disease: Sexual transmission. International Journal of Infectious Diseases. 2019;**81**:81-84. DOI: 10.1016/j.ijid.2019.01.021. Epub 2019 Jan 18

[9] Jackson Y, Pinto A, Pett S. Chagas disease in Australia and New Zealand: Risks and needs for public health interventions. Tropical Medicine & International Health. 2014;**19**:212-218

[10] Norman FF, Lopez-Velez R. Mother-to-child transmission of trypanosoma cruzi infection (chagas disease): A neglected problem. Transactions of the Royal Society of Tropical Medicine and Hygiene. 2014;**108**:388-390

[11] Requena-Mendez A, Albajar-Vinas P, Angheben A, Chiodini P, Gascon J, Munoz J, et al. Health policies to control chagas disease transmission in european countries. PLoS Neglected Tropical Diseases. 2014;**8**:e3245

[12] Velásquez-Ortiz N, Hernández C, Herrera G, Cruz-Saavedra L, Higuera A, Arias-Giraldo LM, et al. *Trypanosoma cruzi* infection, discrete typing units and feeding sources among *Psammolestes arthuri* (reduviidae: Triatominae) collected in eastern Colombia. Parasites & Vectors. 2019;**12**:157

[13] Roca Saumell C, Soriano-Arandes A, Solsona Díaz L, Gascón Brustenga J. Consensus document for the detection and management of chagas disease in primary health care in a non-endemic areas. Grupo de consenso chagas-APS. Atencion Primaria. 2015;**47**(5):308-317

[14] Moure Z, Angheben A, Molina I, Gobbi F, Espasa M, Anselmi M, et al. Serodiscordance in chronic chagas disease diagnosis: A real problem in non-endemic countries. Clinical Microbiology and Infection. 2016;**22**(9):788-792. DOI: 10.1016/j.cmi.2016.06.001. pii: S1198-743X(16)30186-0

[15] Hernández-Hernández FC, Rodríguez MH. Biotechnological advances in infectious diseases diagnosis. Salud Pública de México. 2009;**51**(suppl 3):S424-S438

[16] Peeling RW, Nwaka S. Drugs and diagnostic innovations to improve global health. Infectious Disease Clinics of North America. 2011;**25**:693-705

[17] Romay-Barja M, Boquete T, Martinez O, González M, Álvarez-Del Arco D, Benito A, et al. Chagas screening and treatment among Bolivians living in Madrid, Spain: The need for an official protocol. PLoS One. 2019;**14**(3):e0213577. DOI: 10.1371/journal.pone.0213577

[18] Becerril M. Parasitología Médica. Tercera edición ed. México DF, México: McGraw Hill Interamericana Editores; 2011. pp. 81-93

[19] Guhl F, Vallejo AG. Trypanosoma (herpetosoma) rangeli tejera, 1920—An updated review. Memórias do Instituto Oswaldo Cruz. 2003;**98**:435-442

[20] Reiche EM, Cavazzana M Jr, Okamura H, Tagata EC, Jankevicius SI, Jankevicius JV. Evaluation of the western blot in the confirmatory serologic diagnosis of chagas' disease. The American Journal of Tropical Medicine and Hygiene. 1998;**59**(5):750-756

[21] Escalante H, Jara C, Davelois K, Iglesias M, Benites A, Espinoza R. Western blot technique standardization for specific diagnosis of Chagas disease using excretory-secretory antigens of *Trypanosoma cruzi* epimastigotes. Revista Peruana de Medicina Experimental y Salud Pública. 2014;**31**(4):644-651

[22] Ramos-Ligonio A, Ramírez-Sánchez ME, González-Hernández JC, Rosales-Encina JL, López-Monteon A. Prevalence of antibodies against *Trypanosoma cruzi* in blood bank donors from the IMSS general Hospital in Orizaba, Veracruz, Mexico. Salud Pública de México. 2006;**48**:13-21

[23] Picado A, Cruz I, Redard-Jacot M, et al. The burden of congenital chagas disease and implementation of molecular diagnostic tools in Latin America. BMJ Global Health. 2018;**3**:e001069. DOI: 10.1136/bmjgh-2018-001069

[24] Umezawa ES, Luquetti AO, Levitus G, Ponce C, Ponce E, Henriquez D, et al. Serodiagnosis of chronic and acute Chagas' disease with *Trypanosoma cruzi* recombinant proteins: Results of a collaborative study in six latin american countries. Journal of Clinical Microbiology. 2004;**42**(1):449-452

[25] De Winne K, Büscher P, Luquetti AO, Tavares SB, Oliveira RA, Solari A, et al. The *Trypanosoma cruzi* satellite DNA oligoC-test and *Trypanosoma cruzi* kinetoplast DNA oligoC-test for diagnosis of chagas disease: A multi-cohort comparative evaluation study. PLoS Neglected Tropical Diseases. 2014;**8**:e2633

[26] Portela-Lindoso AA, Shikanai-Yasuda MA. Chronic Chagas' disease: From xenodiagnosis and hemoculture to polymerase chain reaction. Revista de Saúde Pública. 2003;**37**(1):107-115

[27] Schijman AG, Bisio M, Orellana L, Sued M, Duffy T, Mejia Jaramillo AM, et al. International study to evaluate PCR methods for detection of *Trypanosoma cruzi* DNA in blood samples from chagas disease patients. PLoS Neglected Tropical Diseases. 2011;**5**:e931

[28] Ávila H, Pereira J, Thiemmano DE, Paiva E, Degrave W, Morel C, et al. Detection of trypanosoma cruzi in blood specimens of chronic chagasic patients by polymerase chain reaction amplification of kinetoplast minicircle DNA: Comparison with serology and

xenodiagnosis. Journal of Clinical Microbiology. 1993;**31**:2421-2426

[29] Wincker P, Bosseno MF, Britto C, Yaksic N, Cardoso MA, Morel CM, et al. High correlation between chagas disease serology and PCR-based detection of *Trypanosoma cruzi* kinetoplast DNA in bolivian children living in an endemic area. FEMS Microbiology Letters. 1994;**124**(3):419-424

[30] Ferrer E, Da CF, Campioli P, Lares M, López M, Rivera MG, et al. Validación de protocolos de PCR para el diagnóstico molecular de la enfermedad de Chagas. Salus. 2009;**12**(S1):163-174

[31] Perez CJ, Lymbery AJ, Thompson RC. Chagas disease: The challenge of polyparasitism? Trends in Parasitology. 2014;**30**(4):176-182

[32] Ramirez JD, Guhl F, Umezawa ES, Morillo CA, Rosas F, Marin-Neto JA, et al. Evaluation of adult chronic chagas heart disease diagnosis by molecular and serological methods. Journal of Clinical Microbiology. 2009;**47**:3945-3951

[33] Nagarkatti R, de Araujo FF, Gupta C, Debrabant A. Aptamer based, non-PCR, non-serological detection of chagas disease biomarkers in trypanosoma cruzi infected mice. PLoS Neglected Tropical Diseases. 2014;**8**(1):e2650. DOI: 10.1371/journal.pntd.0002650

[34] Wen JJ, Zago MP, Nunez S, Gupta S, Burgos FN, Garg NJ. Serum proteomic signature of human chagasic patients for the identification of novel potential protein biomarkers of disease. Molecular & Cellular Proteomics. 2012;**11**:435-452

[35] Abras A, Gállego M, Llovet T, Tebar S, Herrero M, Berenguer P, et al. Serological diagnosis of chronic chagas disease: Is it time for a change? Journal of Clinical Microbiology. 2016;**54**:1566-1572

[36] Gorlin J, Rossmann S, Robertson G, Stallone F, Hirschler N, Nguyen KA, et al. Evaluation of a new *Trypanosoma cruzi* antibody assay for blood donor screening. Transfusion. 2008;**48**:531-540

[37] Longhi SA, Brandariz SB, Lafon SO, Niborski LL, Luquetti AO, Schijman AG, et al. Evaluation of in-house ELISA using *Trypanosoma cruzi* lysate and recombinant antigens for diagnosis of chagas disease and discrimination of its clinical forms. The American Journal of Tropical Medicine and Hygiene. 2012;**87**:267-271

[38] WHOControl of chagas disease: Second report of the WHO expert committee. World Health Organization Technical Report Series. 2002;**905**:1-109

[39] Viotti R, Vigliano C, Lococo B, Bertocchi G, Petti M, Alvarez MG, et al. Long-term cardiac outcomes of treating chronic chagas disease with benznidazole versus no treatment: A nonrandomized trial. Annals of Internal Medicine. 2006;**144**(10):724-734

[40] Caballero ZC, Sousa OE, Marques WP, Saez-Alquezar A, Umezawa ES. Evaluation of serological tests to identify *Trypanosoma cruzi* infection in humans and determine cross-reactivity with trypanosoma rangeli and leishmania spp. Clinical and Vaccine Immunology. 2007;**14**:1045-1049

[41] Lapa JS, Saraiva RM, Hasslocher-Moreno AM, Georg I, Souza AS, Xavier SS, et al. Dealing with initial inconclusive serological results for chronic chagas disease in clinical practice. European Journal of Clinical Microbiology & Infectious Diseases. 2012;**31**:965-974

[42] Reyes M, Luquetti A, Rassi A, Frasch A. Long lasting IgM and IgG reactivities against *Trypanosoma cruzi*

antigens in human cases of chagas disease. Anales de la Asociacion Quimica Argentina. 1993;**81**:101-110

[43] Andrade S, Freitas L, Peyrol S, Pimentel A, Sadigursky M. Experimental chemotherapy of *Trypanosoma cruzi* infections persistence of parasite antigens and positive serology in parasitologically cured mice. Bulletin of the World Health Organization. 1991;**69**:191-199

[44] Andrade S, Pimentel A, de Souza M, Andrade Z. Interstitial dendritic cells of the Herat harbor *Trypanosoma cruzi* antigens in experimentally infected dogs: Importance for the pathogenesis of chagasic myocarditis. The American Journal of Tropical Medicine and Hygiene. 2000;**63**:64-70

[45] Sosa S, Segura E, Ruiz A, Velásquez E, Porcel B, Yampotis C. Efficacy of chemotherapy with benznidazole in children in the indeterminate phase of chagas´ disease. The American Journal of Tropical Medicine and Hygiene. 1998;**59**:526-529

[46] Andrade A, Zicker F, Oliveira R, Almeida S, Luquetti A, Travassos L, et al. Randomized trial of efficacy of benznidazole in treatment of early *Trypanosoma cruzi* infection. Lancet. 1996;**348**:1407-1413

[47] Cançado J. Criteria of chagas disease cure. Memórias do Instituto Oswaldo Cruz. 1999;**94**(suppl I):331-335

[48] Sanchez Negrette O, Sánchez Valdéz FJ, Lacunza CD, García Bustos MF, Mora MC, Uncos AD, et al. Serological evaluation of specific-antibody levels in patients treated for chronic chagas disease. Clinical and Vaccine Immunology. 2008;**15**:297-302

[49] Ferrer E. Técnicas moleculares para el diagnóstico de la enfermedad de Chagas. SABER. Revista Multidisciplinaria del Consejo de Investigación de la Universidad de Oriente. 2015;**27**:359-371

[50] De Lima A, Arévalo P, Bastidas V, Bolívar M, Navarro M, Contreras V. Efecto de las condiciones de mantenimiento de *Trypanosoma cruzi* sobre la calidad de los antígenos para el diagnóstico serológico de la enfermedad de Chagas. Salus. 2007;**11**(suppl 1): 20-26

[51] Amato-Neto V, De Marchi CR, Ferreira CS, Ferreira AW. Observations on the use of TESA blot for the serological diagnosis of chagas' disease. Revista da Sociedade Brasileira de Medicina Tropical. 2005;**38**:534-535

[52] Chang K, Cheng Y, Jiang LX, Salbilla VA, Haller AS, Yem AW. Evaluation of a prototype *Trypanosoma cruzi* antibody assay with recombinant antigens on a fully automated chemiluminescence analyzer for blood donor screening. Transfusion. 2006;**46**:1737-1744

[53] Flores-Chávez M, Cruz I, Rodríguez M, Nieto J, Franco E, Gárate T, et al. Comparación de técnicas serológicas convencionales y no convencionales para el diagnóstico de la enfermedad de Chagas importada en España. Enfermedades Infecciosas y Microbiología Clínica. 2010;**28**:284-293

[54] Umezawa ES, Nascimento MS, Kesper N Jr, Coura JR, Borges-Pereira J, Junqueira AC. Immunoblot assay using excreted-secreted antigens of *Trypanosoma cruzi* in serodiagnosis of congenital, acute, and chronic chagas' disease. Journal of Clinical Microbiology. 1996;**34**:2143-2147

[55] Wendel S. Transfusion-transmitted american and african trypanosomiasis (chagas disease and sleeping sickness): Neglected or reality? ISBT Science Series. 2006;**1**:140-151

[56] Winkler MA, Brashear RJ, Hall HJ, Schur JD, Pan AA. Detection of

antibodies to trypanosoma cruzi among blood donors in the southwestern and western United States. II. Evaluation of a supplemental enzyme immunoassay and radioimmunoprecipitation assay for confirmation of seroreactivity. Transfusion. 1995;**35**:219-225

[57] Da Silveira JF, Umezawa ES, Luquetti AO. Chagas disease: Recombinant *Trypanosoma cruzi* antigens for serological diagnosis. Trends in Parasitology. 2001;**17**:286-291

[58] Teixeira-Carvalho A, Campos FM, Geiger SM, Rocha RD, de Araújo FF, Vitelli-Avelar DM, et al. FC-TRIPLEX Chagas/Leish IgG1: A multiplexed flow cytometry method for differential serological diagnosis of chagas disease and leishmaniasis. PLoS One. 2015;**e0122938**:10. DOI: 10.1371

[59] Martins-Filho OA, Pereira ME, Carvalho JF, Cançado JR, Brener Z. Flow cytometry, a new approach to detect anti-live trypomastigote antibodies and monitor the efficacy of specific treatment in human Chagas' disease. Clinical and Diagnostic Laboratory Immunology. 1995;**2**(5):569-573

[60] Foti L, Fonseca B d P, Nascimento LD, Marques C d F, da Silva ED, Duarte CA, et al. Viability study of a multiplex diagnostic platform for chagas disease. Memórias do Instituto Oswaldo Cruz. 2009;**104**(Suppl 1):136-141

[61] Luqueti A, Ponce C, Ponce E, Estefandiari J, Schijman A, Revollo S, et al. Chagas disease diagnosis: A multicentric evaluation of Chagas Stat-Pak, a rapid immunocrhromatographic assay with recombinant proteins of *Trypanosoma cruzi*. Diagnostic Microbiology and Infectious Disease. 2003;**46**:265-271

[62] López-Chejade P, Roca C, Posada E, Pinazo MJ, Gascon J, Portús M. Utility of an immunochromatographic test for chagas disease screening in primary healthcare. Enfermedades Infecciosas y Microbiología Clínica. 2010;**28**:169-171

[63] Sánchez-Camargo CL, Albajar-Viñas P, Wilkins PP, Nieto J, Leiby DA, Paris L, et al. Comparative evaluation of 11 commercialized rapid diagnostic tests for detecting *Trypanosoma cruzi* antibodies in serum banks in areas of endemicity and nonendemicity. Journal of Clinical Microbiology. 2014;**54**(7):2506-2512

[64] Oliveira LC, Lee TH, Ferreira AM, Bierrenbach AL, Souza-Basqueira M, Oliveira CDL, et al. Lack of evidence of seronegative infection in an endemic area of chagas disease. Revista do Instituto de Medicina Tropical de São Paulo. 2019;**61**:e11. DOI: 10.1590/S1678-9946201961011

[65] Morocoima A, Socorro G, Avila R, Hernández A, Merchán S, Ortiz D, et al. *Trypanosoma cruzi*: Experimental parasitism in the central nervous system of albino mice. Parasitology Research. 2012;**111**:2099-2107

[66] Tarleton RL, Reithinger R, Urbina JA, Kitron U, Gürtler RE. The challenges of chagas disease—Grim outlook or glimmer of hope. PLoS Medicine. 2007;**4**:e332

[67] Moure Z, Sulleiro E, Iniesta L, Guillen C, Molina I, Alcover MM, et al. The challenge of discordant serology in Chagas disease: The role of two confirmatory techniques in inconclusive cases. Acta Tropica. 2018;**185**:144-148. DOI: 10.1016/j.actatropica.2018.05.010. Epub 2018 May 15

[68] Viotti R, Vigliano C, Alvarez MG, Lococo B, Petti M, Bertocchi G, et al. Impact of aetiological treatment on conventional and multiplex serology in chronic chagas disease. PLoS Neglected Tropical Diseases. 2011;**5**(9):e1314. DOI: 10.1371/journal.pntd.0001314

[69] Guzmán-Gómez D, López-Monteon A, Lagunes-Castro S, Álvarez-Martínez C, Hernández-Lutzon MJ, Dumonteil E, et al. Highly discordant serology against *Trypanosoma cruzi* in Central Veracruz, Mexico: Role of the antigen used for diagnostic. Parasites & Vectors. 2015;**17**(8):466

[70] De Souza RM, Amato V. Discrepancies and consequences of indirect hemagglutination, indirect immunofluorescence and elisa tests for the diagnosis of chagas disease. Revista do Instituto de Medicina Tropical de São Paulo. 2012;**54**:141-143

[71] Santos FL, de Souza WV, Barros Mda S, Nakazawa M, Krieger MA, Gomes Y d M. Chronic chagas disease diagnosis: A comparative performance of commercial enzyme immunoassay tests. American Journal of Tropical Medicine and Hygiene. 2016;**94**(5):1034-1039. DOI: 10.4269/ajtmh.15-0820.

[72] Langhi DM Jr, Bordin JO, Castelo A, Walter SD, Moraes-Souza H, Stumpf RJ. The application of latent class analysis for diagnostic test validation of chronic *Trypanosoma cruzi* infection in blood donors. The Brazilian Journal of Infectious Diseases. 2002;**6**:181-187

[73] Leiby DA, Wendel S, Takaoka DT, Fachini RM, Oliveira LC, Tibbals MA. Serologic testing for *Trypanosoma cruzi*: Comparison of radioimmunoprecipitation assay with commercially available indirect immunofluorescence assay, indirect hemagglutination assay, and enzyme-linked immunosorbent assay kits. Journal of Clinical Microbiology. 2000;**38**:639-642

[74] Otero S, Sulleiro E, Molina I, Espiau M, Suy A, Martín-Nalda A, et al. Congenital transmission of *Trypanosoma cruzi* in non-endemic areas: Evaluation of a screening program in a tertiary care hospital in Barcelona, Spain. The American Journal of Tropical Medicine and Hygiene. 2012;**87**(5):832-836

[75] Carlier Y, Torrico F, Sosa-Estani S, Russomando G, Luquetti A, Freilij H, et al. Congenital chagas disease: Recommendations for diagnosis, treatment and control of newborns, siblings and pregnant women. PLoS Neglected Tropical Diseases. 2011;**5**(10):e1250

[76] Riera C, Verges M, Iniesta L, Fisa R, Gállego M, Tebar S, et al. Identification of a Western blot pattern for the specific diagnosis of *Trypanosoma cruzi* infection in human sera. The American Journal of Tropical Medicine and Hygiene. 2012;**86**:412-416

[77] Torres-Gutiérrez E, Barrios-Palacios D, Ruiz-Hernández AL, Cabrera-Bravo M, Guevara-Gómez Y, Rojas-Wastavino G, et al. Identification of immunodominant components of an isolate of *Trypanosoma cruzi* by immunoblot and its standardization for diagnostic purposes. Gaceta Médica de México. 2015;**151**(1):6-13

[78] Gil j CR, López I, Cajal S, Acosta N, Juarez M, Zacca R, et al. Reactividad del antígeno GST-SAPA de *Trypanosoma cruzi* frente a sueros de pacientes con enfermedad de Chagas y leishmaniasis. Medicina. 2011;**71**:113-119

[79] Otani MM, Vinelli E, Kirchhoff LV, del Pozo A, Sands A, Vercauteren G, et al. WHO. Comparative evaluation of serologic assays for chagas disease. Transfusion. 2009;**49**(6):1076-1082

[80] Silveira-Lacerda EP, Silva AG, Junior SF, Souza MA, Kesper N, Botelho-Filho A, et al. Chagas' disease: Application of TESA-blot in inconclusive sera from a Brazilian blood bank. Vox Sanguinis. 2004;**87**(3):204-207

[81] Umezawa ES, Souza AI, Pinedo-Cancino V, Marcondes M, Marcili A, Camargo LM, et al. TESA-blot for the diagnosis of chagas disease in dogs from co-endemic regions for *Trypanosoma cruzi*, *Trypanosoma evansi* and *Leishmania chagasi*. Acta Tropica. 2009;**111**(1):15-20

[82] Caballero EZ, Correa R, Nascimento MS, Villarreal A, Llanes A, Kesper N Jr. High sensitivity and reproducibility of in-house ELISAs using different genotypes of *Trypanosoma cruzi*. Parasite Immunology. 2019;e12627. https://doi.org/10.1111/pim.12627

[83] Gomes YM, Pereira VR, Nakazawa M, Rosa DS, Barros MD, Ferreira AG. Serodiagnosis of chronic chagas infection by using EIE-recombinant-chagas-biomanguinhos kit. Memórias do Instituto Oswaldo Cruz. 2001;**96**:497-501

[84] Enciso C, Montilla M, Santacruz MM, Nicholls RS, Rodríguez A, Mercado M. Comparison of the indirect immunofluorescent (IFAT), ELISA test and the commercial chagatek test for anti-*Trypanosoma cruzi* antibodies detection. Biomédica. 2004;**24**:104-108

[85] Sánchez B, Monteon V, Reyes PA, Espinoza B. Standardization of micro-enzyme-linked immunosorbent assay (ELISA) and Western blot for detection of *Trypanosoma cruzi* antibodies using extracts from Mexican strains as antigens. Archives of Medical Research. 2001;**32**:382-388

[86] Bosseno MF, Barnabe C, Magallon GE, Lozano KF, Ramsey J, Espinoza B. Predominance of *Trypanosoma cruzi* lineage I in Mexico. Journal of Clinical Microbiology. 2002;**40**:627-632

[87] Miles MA, Feliciangeli MD, De Arias AR. American trypanosomiasis (chagas' disease) and the role of molecular epidemiology in guiding control strategies. BMJ. 2003;**326**:1444-1448

[88] Herrera CP, Licon MH, Nation CS, Jameson SB, Wesson DM. Genotype diversity of *Trypanosoma cruzi* in small rodents and *Triatoma sanguisuga* from a rural area in New Orleans, Louisiana. Parasites & Vectors. 2015;**24, 8**:123

[89] Ramos-Ligonio A, Torres-Montero J, Lopez-Monteon A, Dumonteil E. Extensive diversity of *Trypanosoma cruzi* discrete typing units circulating in Triatoma dimidiata from Central Veracruz, Mexico. Infection, Genetics and Evolution. 2012;**12**(7):1341-1343

[90] Andersson J, Orn A, Sunnemark D. Chronic murine chagas disease: The impact of host and parasite genotypes. Immunology Letters. 2003;**86**:207-212

[91] Macedo AM, Pena SD. Genetic variability of *Trypanosoma cruzi*: Implications for the pathogenesis of chagas disease. Parasitology Today. 1998;**14**:119-124

[92] Zingales B, Miles MA, Campbell DA, Tibayrenc M, Macedo AM, Teixeira MM, et al. The revised trypanosoma cruzi subspecific nomenclature: Rationale, epidemiological relevance and research applications. Infection, Genetics and Evolution. 2012;**12**:240-253

[93] Houghton RL, Benson DR, Reynolds L, McNeill P, Sleath P, Lodes M, et al. Multiepitope synthetic peptide and recombinant protein for the detection of antibodies to *Trypanosoma cruzi* in patients with treated or untreated Chagas' disease. The Journal of Infectious Diseases. 2000;**181**(1):325-330

[94] Umezawa ES, Bastos SF, Coura JR, Levin MJ, Gonzalez A, Rangel-Aldao R, et al. An improved serodiagnostic test for chagas' disease employing a mixture

of *Trypanosoma cruzi* recombinant antigens. Transfusion. 2003;**43**:91-97

[95] Alvarez P, Leguizamo'n MS, Buscaglia CA, Pitcovsky TA, Campetella O. Multiple overlapping epitopes in the repetitive unit of the shed acute-phase antigen from *Trypanosoma cruzi* enhance its immunogenic properties. Infection and Immunity. 2001;**69**:7946-7949

[96] Vanniasinkam T, Barton MD, Heuzenroeder MW. B-cell epitope mapping of the VapA protein of *Rhodococcus equi*: Implications for early detection of *R. equi* disease in foals. Journal of Clinical Microbiology. 2001;**39**:1633-1637

[97] Andresen H, Bier FF. Peptide microarrays for serum antibody diagnostics. Methods in Molecular Biology. 2009;**509**:123-134

[98] Pellois JP, Zhou X, Srivannavit O, Zhou T, Gulari E, Gao X. Individually addressable parallel peptide synthesis on microchips. Nature Biotechnology. 2002;**20**:922-926

[99] Carmona SJ, Sartor PA, MS L'n, Campetella OE, Agüero F. Diagnostic peptide discovery: Prioritization of pathogen diagnostic markers using multiple features. PLoS One. 2012;**7**(12):e50748

[100] Carmona SJ, Nielsen M, Schafer-Nielsen C, Mucci J, Altcheh J, Balouz V, et al. Towards high-throughput immunomics for infectious diseases: Use of next-generation peptide microarrays for rapid discovery and mapping of antigenic determinants. Molecular & Cellular Proteomics. 2015;**14**:1871-1884

[101] Larsen JEP, Lund O, Nielsen M. Improved method for predicting linear B-cell epitopes. Immunome Res. 2006;**24**:2-9

[102] Liang S, Zheng D, Standley DM, Yao B, Zacharias M, Zhang C. EPSVR and EPMeta: Prediction of antigenic epitopes using support vector regression and multiple server results. BMC Bioinformatics. 2010;**11**:381

[103] Ponomarenko J, Bui HH, Li W, Fusseder N, Bourne PE, Sette A, et al. ElliPro: A new structure-based tool for the prediction of antibody epitopes. BMC Bioinformatics. 2008;**9**:514

[104] Sweredoski MJ, Baldi P. PEPITO: Improved discontinuous B-cell epitope prediction using multiple distance thresholds and half sphere exposure. Bioinformatics. 2008;**24**:1459-1460

[105] Sweredoski MJ, Baldi P. COBEpro: A novel system for predicting continuous B-cell epitopes. Protein Engineering, Design & Selection. 2009;**22**:113-120

[106] Ekins R, Chu FW. Microarrays: Their origins and applications. Trends in Biotechnology. 1999;**17**:217-218

[107] Wilson DS, Nock S. Recent developments in protein microarray technology. Angewandte Chemie (International Ed. in English). 2003;**42**(5):494-500

[108] Almeida IC, Covas DT, Soussumi LM, Travassos LR. A highly sensitive and specific chemiluminescent enzyme-linked immunosorbent assay for diagnosis of active *Trypanosoma cruzi* infection. Transfusion. 1997;**37**:850-857

[109] De Marchi CR, Di Noia JM, Frasch ACC, Amato Neto V, Almeida IC, Buscaglia CA. Evaluation of a recombinant *Trypanosoma cruzi* mucin-like antigen for serodiagnosis of chagas' disease. Clinical and Vaccine Immunology. 2011;**18**:1850-1855

[110] Faraudo S, López N, Canela B, Guimarães A, Sáez-Alquezar

A. Evaluation in Brazil of the new bio-flash chagas assay on Biokit's bio-flash analyzer. Revista Española de Salud Pública. 2015:65-66

[111] Imaz-Iglesia I, Miguel LGS, Ayala-Morillas LE, García-Pérez L, González-Enríquez J, Blasco-Hernández T, et al. Economic evaluation of chagas disease screening in Spain. Acta Tropica. 2015;**148**:77-88

[112] Lee BY, Bacon KM, Bottazzi ME, Hotez PJ. Global economic burden of chagas disease: A computational simulation model. The Lancet Infectious Diseases. 2013;**13**:342-348

[113] Ramsey JM, Elizondo-Cano M, Sanchez-González G, Peña-Nieves A, Figueroa-Lara A. Opportunity cost for early treatment of chagas disease in Mexico. PLoS Neglected Tropical Diseases. 2014;**8**:e2776

[114] Sicuri E, Muñoz J, Pinazo MJ, Posada E, Sanchez J, Alonso PL, et al. Economic evaluation of Chagas disease screening of pregnant Latin American women and of their infants in a non-endemic area. Acta Tropica. 2011;**118**:110-117

[115] Ballesteros GR, Cuevas TIM, Jiménez BR, et al. Chagas disease: An overview of diagnosis. Journal of Microbiology & Experimentation. 2018;**6**(3):151-157. DOI: 10.15406/jmen.2018.06.00207

[116] Ndao M, Spithill TW, Caffrey R, Li H, Podust VN, Perichon R, et al. Identification of novel diagnostic serum biomarkers for Chagas' disease in asymptomatic subjects by mass spectrometric profiling. Journal of Clinical Microbiology. 2010;**48**:1139-1149

[117] De Araujo FF, Vitelli-Avelar DM, Teixeira-Carvalho A, Antas PR, Assis Silva Gomes J, Sathler-Avelar R, et al. Regulatory T cells phenotype in different clinical forms of Chagas' disease. PLoS Neglected Tropical Diseases. 2011;**5**:e992

[118] Adamczyk M, Brashear RJ, Mattingly PG. Circulating cardiac troponin-I autoantibodies in human plasma and serum. Annals of the New York Academy of Sciences. 2009;**1173**:67-74

Chapter 6

Epidemiology of Leprosy in Vietnam and the Effectiveness of Multidrug Therapy (MDT) in the Management of the Disease

Tran Hau Khang, Ngo Minh Thao and Le Huu Doanh

Abstract

Leprosy is a chronic infection caused by the acid-fast, rod-shaped bacillus *Mycobacterium leprae*. Leprosy can be considered connected diseases that primarily affect the superficial tissues, especially the skin and peripheral nerves. The social and psychological effects of leprosy, as well as its highly visible debilities and sequelae, have resulted in a historical stigma associated with leprosy. Vietnam has seen a highly significant decrease in the prevalence rate (PR) of leprosy since 1983. From 1983 onwards, with the introduction of multidrug therapy (MDT), the prevalence of the disease has dropped to less than one case per 10,000 individuals from 1995. After over two decades, a total of 109 cases were registered with a prevalence rate of 0.01 per 10,000 population in 2017. It is clear that over the past 35 years, the profile of leprosy in Vietnam has been changed significantly followed by the treatment with MDT. Leprosy has become a rare disease in Vietnam. This chapter presents the trend in the epidemiology of leprosy in Vietnam from 1983 to 2018 and also mentions the effectiveness of multidrug therapy (MDT) in the management of this disease. Based on individual records and annual reports, the prevalence of registered cases, the number of new cases detected yearly, their sex, age, classification (MB, multibacillary; PB, paucibacillary) and disability status are carefully presented.

Keywords: leprosy, multidrug therapy, relapse, prevalence, incidence, disability

1. Introduction

Vietnam, officially the Socialist Republic of Vietnam, is the easternmost country on the Indochina Peninsula which is a part of the Western Pacific Region. With another four countries, including China, Malaysia, Papua New Guinea and the Philippines, Vietnam contributed to 86% of the total prevalence, according to the WHO's report in 2010 [1]. While the lack of knowledge about leprosy in the lower socio-economic group is an important cause why most of patients with untreated leprosy end up with severe deformities and disfigurements, there has been a degree of stagnation and new approaches in leprosy control. Therefore, in 1991, the global leprosy control network was established. The WHO set the goal of elimination of leprosy as a public health problem in which the prevalence rate needs to be below one case per 10,000 people [2]. Vietnam has achieved the national target in 1995 and succeeded in maintaining the elimination threshold, reaching that sub-nation at the end of the year 2000 [3]. However, based on the annual data collected from 2000 onwards, several new case detections have been reported [3, 4]. This requires continuing the implementation of the main principles of leprosy control in the nation, with a special focus on the five fields, such as timely detection of new cases, contact investigation, multidrug therapy (MDT) treatment, the treatment compliance and prevention of disabilities and also rehabilitation. The strategic directions are integration, early diagnosis and treatment which help to strengthen and sustain leprosy activities, quality patient care and reduction of the leprosy burden of physical, social and economic consequences. The introduction of MDT for the treatment of leprosy in 1983 was one of the important landmarks in combating the disease. In the past, many clinical trials of MDT have been implemented with high effectiveness and well toleration. The addition of ofloxacin to multidrug regimens has been developed to reduce the required duration of MDT possible. Moderate to marked clinical and bacterial improvement with minimal adverse effects has been observed [5, 6].

2. Network of leprosy control programme

Vietnam's National Leprosy Control Programme was established in 1982 [7]. The present national framework for leprosy control is characterized by the integrated delivery of basic leprosy services, which are provided at the peripheral level. The leprosy control system is a part of the healthcare system which follows the administrative system (**Figure 1**). The National Hospital of Dermatology and Venereology (NHDV) is the leading institute responsible to the Ministry of Health (MOH) for skin diseases, sexually transmitted infections (STIs) and leprosy control in the

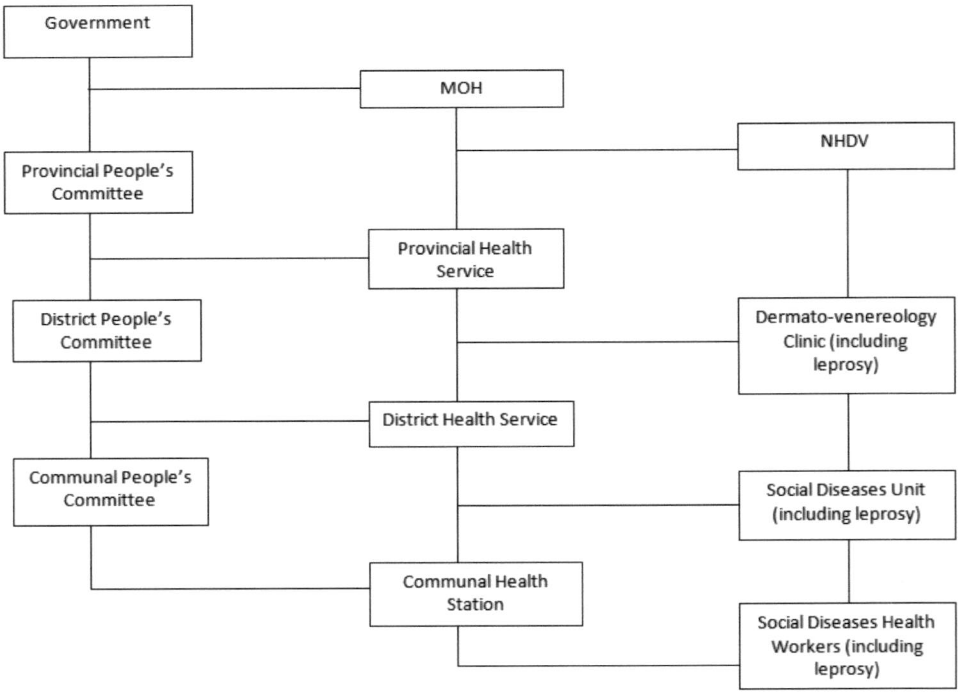

Figure 1.
Leprosy control system according to healthcare and administrative system.

whole country [4]. There are the supported systems, namely, Dermato-Venereology Clinic, vertically under NHDV in each province, covering these fields at provincial level. Dermato-venereological activities including leprology work are continuously separated into the leprosy programmes at district level. At the district's social diseases unit in endemic zones, several practitioners are specially trained to work exclusively in leprosy field, whereas in less endemic district, they are in charge of some contagious diseases, including leprosy, tuberculosis, malaria, HIV/AIDS, etc. In each commune that includes 2–5 villages with 1000–3000 people, leprosy and other social diseases are managed by one or two health workers. They are the specialized units with leprosy expertise at intermediate levels that provide the necessary technical guidance. Their main work is to refer suspect cases for diagnosis confirmation, to treat and to follow up confirmed cases. Antileprosy drugs are stored at any levels, from central to local. The leprosy programme plays a paramount importance to facilitate early case detection and reduce the disease burden further in all endemic areas because they encourage voluntary or self-reporting and help increase the capabilities of the peripheral general healthcare staff through training.

3. Epidemiology of leprosy

3.1 Before 1975

There is no exact data of this period because dermato-venereology profession network was just established in 1975, but the estimated prevalence rate of leprosy was 6–7/10,000 population in 1975 [4]. Most of patients are being congregated in places such as leprosy villages/colonies despite no segregation law.

3.2 From 1976 to 2018

The National Leprosy Control Programme (NLCP) was formed in 1982, and MDT was implemented 1 year later, in 1983 [7].

3.2.1 The trend in prevalence rate of leprosy

According to the annual data reported from 1983 to 2018, there was a decreasing trend in both prevalence rate and the annual newly detected cases (**Figure 2**). As a result of the long-term efforts, Vietnam, which was one of the first 15 countries in the region, had reached the goal of elimination at the national level in 1995 with the prevalence rate of 0.7 per 10,000 population [2]. At the end of the year 2000, the subnational target has been reported. In 2000, only 28 provinces reached Vietnam's 3 elimination criteria [3, 4]. But from 2001 to 2015, all the rest 36 provinces completed the WHO's elimination goal at the provincial level in the country (Vietnam's 4 elimination criteria) [7], and relatively high case detection rate was found in some area, particularly in the central highland and some southern provinces.

They were varied from 38,652 prevalent cases in 1983, corresponding a rate of 6.78 per 10,000 people, to 18,418 cases, corresponding of 2.71 in 1991 (see **Table 1**). During this period, the registered prevalence number was very high due to several main factors, such as retreated with MDT in patients previously treated with dapsone and managing the national leprosy by using 24-month regimen without ofloxacin. However, since 1992 onwards, the number of registered prevalence cases reduced dramatically (**Figure 2**). Starting from 9245 cases in 1992, it decreased to 96 in 2018 and the rate dropped continuously from 1.36 to 0.01 per 10,000

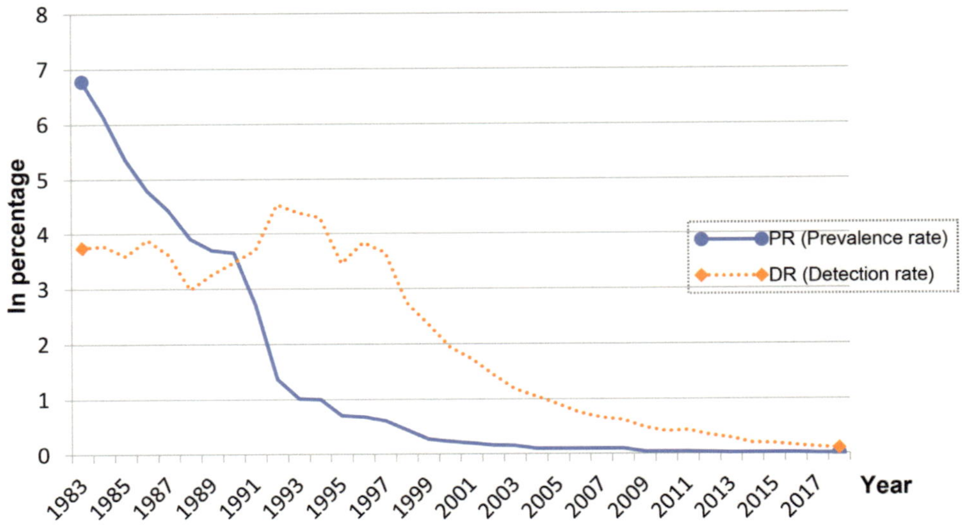

Figure 2.
Prevalence rate (PR) and detection rate (DR) of leprosy (1983–2018) (detection rate (DR), proportion of new cases per 100,000 population; prevalence rate (PR), proportion of leprosy cases per 10,000 population).

population in the same period (**Table 1**). The main reasons were considered, such as disseminating MDT therapy in the whole country and introducing patients to 12-month regimen for shortening the required duration of MDT possible in 1998.

Analysis of a total data from 1983 to 2018 revealed that the prevalence rate has dropped significantly from 6.78 per 10,000 in 1983 to 0.01 per 10,000 in 2018 (**Table 1**). It is clear that over the past 35 years, the prevalence rate of leprosy has changed dramatically by around 99.9%. With this prevalence rate, it was believed that the transmission of *M. leprae* would be reduced and leprosy would naturally disappear. The post-elimination challenges in the future are sustaining high-quality leprosy programmes and reaching the target of district level. Although leprosy has become a rare disease in Vietnam, all activities of the NLCP are sustained from the national to grassroot levels. At the present, Vietnam has several provinces which achieved the goal of elimination at the district level.

3.2.2 Trend in case detection

The new cases include patients who are newly diagnosed during the calendar year. Due to the development of the leprosy network and acceleration of activities of health education, the number of new cases detected yearly was remarkably increased from 1991 to 1997 (**Figure 2**). A total of more than 32 special projects, namely, SAPEL, LEC and mini-LEC, were conducted in this period, during 1991–1997 [3]. The results, not only the new case detections but also the remaining undetected cases, especially in the high plateau areas and some places in southern provinces, were found out. During 1993–1998 the number of new cases detected annually increased. From 1999 up to now, the annual detection rate has declined (**Figure 2**). Only 77 cases were detected in 2018 with a rate of 0.1 per 100,000 inhabitants and a decrease from 1795 cases in 1999, corresponding to a rate of 2.35 per 100,000 population (**Table 1**). Compared with other countries in the region, Vietnam has significantly declined in the incidence cases. Between 2013 and 2014, while India alone accounted for 58.85% of the global Leprosy burden, with a total of 127,000 new cases detected, that number in Vietnam was only 521 new cases [8], <243.7 times. Because case detection is highly influenced by the intensity of

Year	Prevalence		Cases detected	
	n	Per 10,000	n	Per 100,000
1983	38,652	6.78	2021	3.74
1984	36,226	6.14	2103	3.77
1985	32,483	5.36	2062	3.59
1986	29,219	4.79	2292	3.88
1987	27,401	4.42	2183	3.61
1988	24,570	3.90	1847	2.98
1989	23,612	3.69	2073	3.26
1990	24,081	3.65	1995	3.47
1991	18,418	2.71	2500	3.69
1992	9245	1.36	3142	4.53
1993	7090	1.01	3185	4.38
1994	7104	1.00	3173	4.29
1995	5277	0.70	2591	3.45
1996	4827	0.68	2883	3.83
1997	4665	0.61	2808	3.65
1998	3482	0.44	2162	2.74
1999	2087	0.27	1795	2.35
2000	1718	0.23	1477	1.94
2001	1532	0.2	1336	1.73
2002	1269	0.16	1158	1.44
2003	1204	0.15	949	1.18
2004	828	0.1	858	1.04
2005	642	0.1	746	0.9
2006	572	0.1	666	0.75
2007	510	0.1	552	0.66
2008	540	0.1	530	0.62
2009	350	0.04	413	0.48
2010	318	0.04	359	0.41
2011	322	0.04	374	0.43
2012	265	0.03	296	0.34
2013	260	0.02	294	0.29
2014	187	0.02	227	0.2
2015	178	0.02	168	0.19
2016	138	0.02	153	0.15
2017	109	0.01	112	0.12
2018	96	0.01	77	0.1

Table 1.
Prevalence and case detection in Vietnam (1983–2018).

programme activities, such as service coverage, community awareness and the reporting system as well as sensitivity and specificity of diagnosis, the new case detection rate may not represent the true incidence and the degree of transmission of infection in the community.

3.2.3 Grade 2 disability proportion among new cases

Leprosy usually affects the skin and peripheral nerves. Visible disability, expressed as grade 2 disabilities, may be noted as the results of involvement damage of certain peripheral nerves [6, 7]. The proportion of grade 2 disabilities among new cases from 1983 to 2018 fluctuated a lot depending on the trend in case detection (see **Figure 3**). The highest rate was 40.82% in 1983 then decreased to 17.86% in 1993 (**Table 2**). The main cause may be related to shortening of timely diagnosis and treatment of cases, before nerve damage has occurred. Ensuring good treatment compliance of patients also led to reduce the visible disability rate. This decline reflected the efficacy of leprosy control activities. The grade 2 disability proportion between 1994 and 1997 increased related to the intensive case-finding efforts that were carried out in this period. The projects including LECs, mini-LECs and SAPEL have detected a large number of backlog cases, most of whom could suffer severe deformities and disfigurements as a result of delayed diagnosis. Additionally, some of old patients re-registered as new cases especially those with disabilities that also contributed to increasing the grade 2 disability proportion among new cases. On the other side, the high stigma and low awareness about the disease in the society

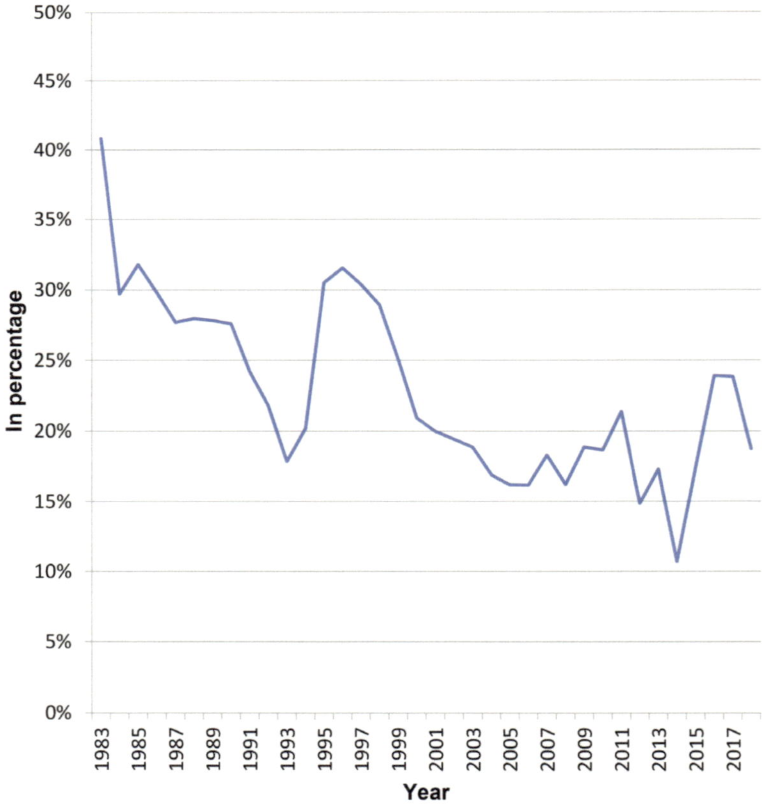

Figure 3.
Proportion of grade 2 disability among new cases.

Year	Grade 2 disabilities	
	Number	Proportion (%)
1983	825	40.82
1984	625	29.70
1985	655	31.77
1986	683	29.80
1987	605	27.70
1988	517	27.99
1989	577	27.83
1990	551	27.62
1991	606	24.20
1992	685	21.80
1993	569	17.86
1994	641	20.20
1995	789	30.50
1996	909	31.53
1997	854	30.40
1998	626	28.95
1999	450	25.07
2000	309	20.92
2001	267	19.99
2002	225	19.43
2003	179	18.86
2004	145	16.90
2005	121	16.22
2006	108	16.20
2007	101	18.30
2008	86	16.23
2009	78	18.89
2010	67	18.66
2011	80	21.39
2012	44	14.86
2013	45	17.31
2014	20	10.7
2015	31	17.42
2016	33	23.91
2017	26	23.85
2018	18	18.75

Table 2.
Proportion of grade 2 disabilities among new cases (1983–2018).

Year	Female		Children under 15 years old		MB cases	
	Number	Proportion (%)	Number	Proportion (%)	Number	Proportion (%)
1983	612	30.28	169	8.59	811	40.10
1984	622	29.50	83	3.95	651	31.13
1985	504	24.40	141	7.84	804	39.10
1986	646	28.20	185	8.07	802	35.20
1987	642	29.40	157	7.21	1009	46.24
1988	509	27.60	141	7.63	738	39.60
1989	466	22.50	120	5.79	932	45.56
1990	463	23.20	130	6.52	798	39.40
1991	494	19.80	120	4.96	1075	43.40
1992	739	23.50	241	7.67	1413	45.50
1993	1114	35.00	231	7.25	1496	47.20
1994	872	27.50	151	4.76	2062	65.20
1995	926	35.70	222	9.57	1632	62.68
1996	1017	35.20	211	7.32	1807	63.70
1997	1011	36.00	159	6.66	1687	59.11
1998	803	37.10	162	6.49	1189	54.67
1999	676	37.70	124	6.91	1071	61.27
2000	571	38.70	105	7.11	905	62.00
2001	497	37.00	77	6.00	822	61.74
2002	437	37.74	65	5.61	715	62.17
2003	339	35.72	52	5.48	616	65.27
2004	322	37.53	47	5.48	570	66.59
2005	269	36.06	39	5.30	492	66.71
2006	245	36.79	35	5.26	443	66.80
2007	178	32.25	25	4.53	377	68.30
2008	202	38.11	18	3.40	378	71.32
2009	144	34.87	12	2.91	295	71.43
2010	98	27.30	14	3.90	259	72.14
2011	121	32.35	11	2.94	269	71.93
2012	105	35.47	10	3.38	191	64.53
2013	82	31.54	14	5.38	180	69.23
2014	66	35.29	7	3.74	153	81.82
2015	53	29.78	5	2.81	143	80.34
2016	39	28.26	4	2.90	115	83.33
2017	38	34.86	2	1.83	91	83.49
2018	24	25.00	0	0	89	92.71

Table 3.
Proportions of female and children in MB patients among newly detected cases (1983–2018).

have contributed to the delay in case detection that affected high grade 2 disability proportion. Fortunately, the rate decreased again and reached a level of 18.75% in 2018 (**Table 2**). It requires that the healthcare system conduct retraining courses on leprosy at provincial, district and communal levels to sustain the effectiveness of the network of leprosy control programme for self-reporting and early treatment.

3.2.4 Female and children among new cases

The age-old stigma associated with the disease remains at least hundreds of years ago in Vietnam. The impact of stigmata attached to leprosy had effect not only on male but also on female and children [7]. Because of the fear of infecting the family members and being divorced, leprosy women were forced to be infertilized and kept themselves aloof. In the past, the children who were born by parental leprosy were not allowed to attend or study with other "normal" children. **Table 3** shows that the distribution of sex and age leprosy patients among new cases was not stable. The proportion of female leprosy detected from 1983 to 2018 was around 19.8–38% (**Figure 4**). This is convenient with other previous studies in some countries in the region such as Thailand, India and Myanmar [1, 2, 8–12].

Here the reported rate of children among new case detection decreased from 169 in 1983 to under 10 cases since 2014 (**Table 3**). From 9.57% in 2000, there is no case observed in 2018 (**Figure 4**). This is a good signal and could be related to success in completing the subnational target at the end of the year 2000 in Vietnam. Some tests have been conducted to make prognosis in high-risk children group, such as gelatin particle agglutination test (GPAT). This measurement tool helped dermatologists to easily assess the transmission of the disease in the community. Tran Hau Khang et al. reported that children with GPAT positive at high titer of more than 1:64 and whose mother/father is a leprosy patient can be considered as the highest risk group developing the disease [13]. As a result, GPAT has proven its important role in early detection of leprosy in children. This could partially explain why the decrease of transmission of the disease led to the reduction in the proportion of children among new cases.

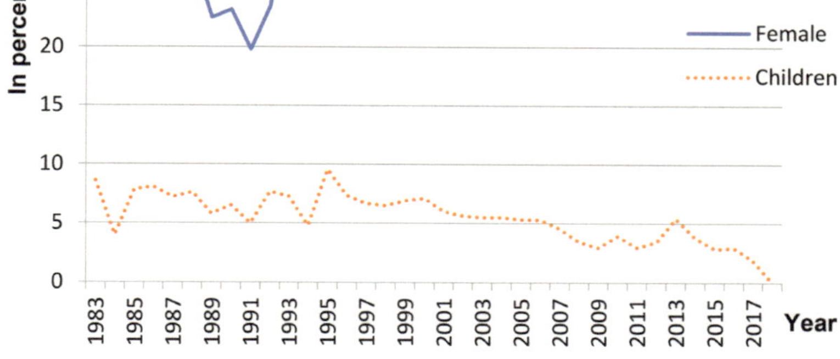

Figure 4.
Proportion of female and children among new cases.

3.2.5 Multibacillary (MB) among new cases

The proportion of MB leprosy among new cases is an important indicator of the magnitude of a potential source of transmission and risk for complications including reactions and neuritis that could lead to disabilities when not treated adequately. In Vietnam, there was the gradual elevation of MB patient rate among newly detected cases from 40.1% in 1983 to 47.2% in 1993. However, from 1994 onwards, the proportion increased significantly. More than 90% (92.71% in 2018) of new case detection were MB patients (**Table 3**). This could be explained by some factor, such as change in the criteria for classification and in the clinical presentations to some extent. Further studies in various countries in the long term are necessary to determine the relation between the operational and the epidemiological factors that are contributing to the increase in MB proportion.

4. Special leprosy projects

In order to enhance knowledge about leprosy which increases misconceptions about the disease's transmission and treatment and to widen case-finding activities in certain areas, several special projects were carried out, such as SAPEL, LECs, mini-LECs and health educational campaigns. A total of 32 activities were implemented from 1991 to 1997 covering over 3 million inhabitants. It comprised 8 LEC projects (1,100,200 populations), 6 SAPEL activities (872,000 individuals) and 18 other activities (1,030,000 people). The number of new cases detected was reported corresponding to these projects: 603, 154 and 663 cases [3, 7]. The total number of newly detected cases in 7 years (1991–1997) was 1420 related to these activities, corresponding to 7% out of total new cases in this period (20,282 cases). This reflected the effectiveness of the network of leprosy control programme. Besides that, the support of the Pacific Leprosy Foundation (PLF) as a partner member and the coordination meetings about leprosy activities that were held with government and local nongovernmental organizations (NGOs) assisted the strengthening of the national leprosy programmes in Vietnam. This ensured programme sustainability by promoting integration within the general health system and also emphasized the need for building and maintaining effective partnerships to improve quality leprosy services and reduce further the disease burden due to leprosy.

5. Effectiveness of MDT in management of leprosy

Leprosy is a long-lasting infection caused by bacteria that can be eliminated by antibiotics. Early diagnosis and treatment of cases can prevent or minimize the onset of further disabilities related to complications, including reactions and neuritis [5, 6, 14–17]. MDT implementation began in 1985 in the Western Pacific Region. It reached 10% coverage in 1988. By 1994, almost 100% MDT coverage was reached [1, 2, 9, 14]. Development and implementation of MDT was the most important achievement in the history of leprosy control in which the introduction of a single-dose treatment regimen for single lesion and 1 year duration for MB leprosy has contributed a great benefit to leprosy patients by shortening of the required duration of MDT. One of the most essential components of the leprosy programme is also ensuring that all new patients who start MDT complete the full course of treatment within the prescribed period of time. A completed treatment patient means that a PB leprosy patient completes 6 monthly doses of PB-MDT within 9 months and a MB leprosy patient completes 12 monthly doses of MB-MDT within 18 months [1, 2, 5, 6, 9, 14]. Vietnam was one of many countries selected as a centre to perform the clinical trial of treatment of leprosy with ofloxacin containing combined drug regimens [5]. Both PB and MB patients undergo six new multidrug regimens containing ofloxacin in comparison with the standard WHO/MDT. The efficacy, tolerance and adverse side effects were considered.

The patients were diagnosed and classified based on bacteriological and clinical manifestations. Both MB and PB patients were randomly allocated to six regimens from A to F. All were examined and followed by the health worker. Individuals were seen daily in the first month and monthly during 5 consecutive months for PB and 23 consecutive months for MB. At the end of treatment, they were assessed once every 6 months for clinical change or any symptom of relapse for at least 10 years.

The results of this previous study showed that all patients treated with ofloxacin-containing regimens have reached moderate to marked clinical and bacterial improvement. However, relapse rate was very high among patients treated with regimen combining ofloxacin and rifampicin daily for 1 month [5, 6]. Several

Year	Complete MDT cases	Implement MDT cases
1995	3460	5277
1996	2831	4527
1997	2669	4665
1998	3229	3482
1999	3060	2077
2000	1820	1718
2001	1478	3044
2002	1362	2740
2003	1042	2258
2004	1209	2102
2005	943	1601
2006	768	1352
2007	640	1159
2008	528	1072
2009	604	976
2010	398	717
2011	339	662
2012	357	622
2013	294	519
2014	227	408
2015	168	342
2016	153	305
2017	112	246
2018	77	203

Table 4.
Number of patients who completed MDT (1995–2018).

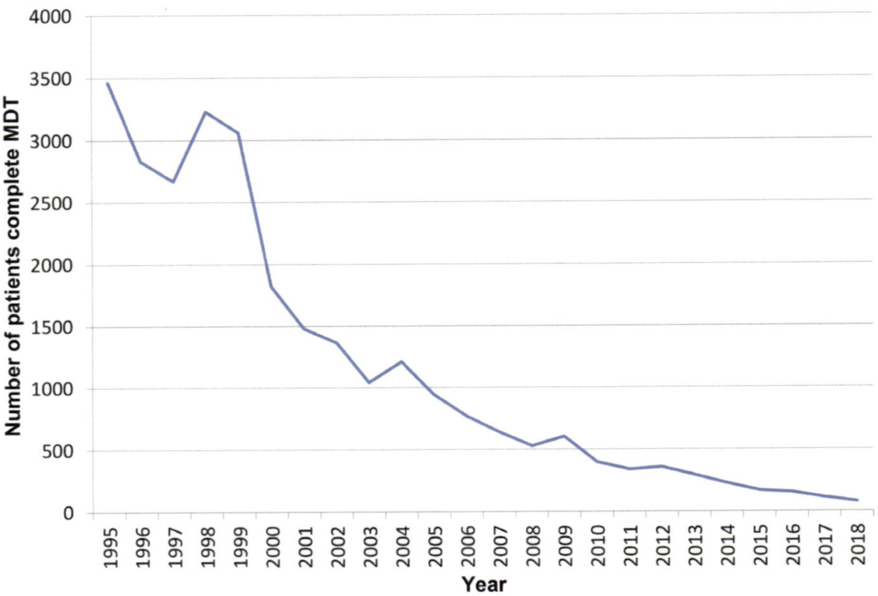

Figure 5.
Number of patients who completed MDT (1995–2018).

adverse side effects were observed, including itch, erythema and vomit, all of which resolved quickly within 2–3 days. Only 1.7% developed erythroderma and required hospitalization [5, 6, 15–17]. With these results, ofloxacin has proven to be a powerful bactericidal drug against *M. leprae*. The introduction of MDT therapy containing Ofloxacin reduced the prevalence rate down to under 0.5% since 1998.

High rate of MB leprosy treatment completion was reported. Nearly 24,000 patients implemented MDT with the completion rate of 100% from 2013 to 2018 (112/112 detected cases treated with MDT in 2017, 77/77 in 2018) (see **Tables 1** and **4**). It coincided with a continuous decline in the prevalence rate (see **Figures 2** and **5**). These results represent the effectiveness of expending efforts of healthcare system form national to grassroot levels. With the financial aid of the government, NGOs and WHO, leprosy patients are treated free of charge with MDT at their own home and can pursue a job suitable to their health. There is lack of data of relapse case during the conduct of MDT therapy from 2000 until now and therefore, the effectiveness of MDT in the management of leprosy in Vietnam over the recent 18 years could not exactly be concluded.

6. Conclusions

With the introduction of MDT in 1983 and the efficacy of leprosy programme activities, the epidemiology of leprosy in Vietnam has dramatically improved. Leprosy is becoming a part of skin neglected tropical diseases (NTDs), a diverse group of communicable diseases that prevail in tropical and subtropical countries, particularly in the easternmost country, Vietnam. At present, leprosy is one of 20 diseases formally recognized as NTDs worldwide. However, three out of five main strategies given to combat NTDs are particularly for leprosy. This means that even though leprosy is considered to be eliminated, the health system including the Ministry of Health and the leading institute, NHDV, in Vietnam are still focusing on sustaining quality leprosy services. Nowadays, majority of the patients are now able to live normal lives in the community without being stigmatized and discriminated. MDT is still the cornerstone of the leprosy control programme in which the timely and regular supply of MDT and proper MDT drug management is very important in attaining the goal of sustaining quality leprosy services and further reducing the leprosy burden. Since 1995, the WHO has supplied MDT free of cost to leprosy patients in all endemic countries. Currently, with the efforts of leprosy network activities, all patients are receiving MDT free from local health facilities.

To maintain these great results, Vietnam set up the Vietnamese criteria for elimination of leprosy at subnational levels including province and district grade since 1997. From three criteria at the beginning, the Ministry of Health decided to set up to five criteria in 2002 [7], such as ensuring that the prevalent proportion in 3 consecutive years is below 0.2 cases per 10,000 people, that the newly detected case rate is under 1 per 100,000 populations and also that the grade 2 disability proportion among new cases is below 15% at the time of examination. The supply criteria were being added to ensure elevating the capacity of health staff worker. There was about 20% of total commune officers, who were randomly checked, who could correctly answer all the content of elimination of leprosy programme. In the future, all activities of the leprosy control programme need to be sustained at all levels, from the nation to the grassroot. With the introduction of the newly detected species of *Mycobacterium*, *Mycobacterium lepromatosis*, in both of MB and PB patients in Mexico in 2008, early detection of *Mycobacterium* which induces leprosy could be a challenge [18, 19]. Further serological tools and other tests on leprosy need to be developed in health service to identify, sequence and detect genes responsible for drug resistance of *Mycobacteria* [20, 21]. In recent years, a few studies in development to investigate the feasibility of a uniform multidrug therapy (U-MDT) regimen for PB and MB patients, with a fixed duration of 6 months, were recommended at the WHO's Technical Advisory Committee meeting in 2002 [22]. China, India, Bangladesh and Brazil were the first four countries performing U-MDT regimen [23–26]. The results showed that there was no statistical difference between the group that received WHO-MDT and those who received U-MDT and also in MB and or PB patients on the frequency of the first reaction occurrence, the mean reduction of BI and the recurrent rates [24–27]. However, in a controlled clinical study in India, from 2003 to 2005, it was observed that for MB patients, U-MDT regimen is not as effective as WHO-MDT with a 12-month duration [23]. Some difficulties related to the disease complexity, clinical trial development and in reproducing the in vitro findings in clinical practice are the obstacles to make the U-MDT regimen accessible to most patients. To this date, there is nothing in short period of time to replace MDT [28]. Recently, the recommendation of the WHO about the implementation of U-MDT among central strategies for leprosy control in the quadrennium 2017/2020 was published [29, 30]. In Vietnam, there was no controlled clinical study, comparing the efficacy of U-MDT and WHO-MDT for PB and MB patients. This advocates the need for new studies to access the effectiveness of U-MDT or new therapeutical regimens in the treatment and management of leprosy in the long term in Vietnam. Thenceforth, all endemic areas have the uniform regimen in the treatment and management of leprosy to sustain the disease in skin NTDs in the long run.

Conflict of interest

No conflict of interest.

Author details

Tran Hau Khang*, Ngo Minh Thao and Le Huu Doanh
National Hospital of Dermatology and Venereology, Hanoi Medical University, Hanoi, Vietnam

*Address all correspondence to: khangquocduc@fpt.vn

References

[1] World Health Organization. Epidemiological Review of leprosy in the Western pacific Region 2008-2010: Sustaining leprosy services and further reducing the leprosy burden. WHO/WPR, Manilar 2010. Available from: https://apps.who.int/iris/handle/10665/207500

[2] World Health Organization. A Guide to Eliminating Leprosy as a Public Health Problem. WHO reference number: WHO/LEP/97

[3] Khang TH. Epidemiology of leprosy in Vietnam, 1983-2012. International Research on Medical Sciences. 2017;**5**:008-015

[4] Pham DB, Koichi S, Norihisa I, et al. Leprosy situation in Vietnam-reduced burden of stigma. Japanese Journal of Leprosy. 2008;**77**:29-36

[5] Tran HK, Vijaykamar P, Pham HL. Treatment of leprosy with ofloxacin-containing combined drug regimens in Vietnam. Vietnamese Journal of Dermatology and Venereology. 2016;**9**:6-14

[6] Due LK, Khang TH. National guidelines for treatment of leprosy with ofloxacin. Vietnamese Journal of Dermatology and Venereology. 1992;**2**:1-18

[7] Ngoan THL. Leprosy. Medical Publishing House; 2002:11-18

[8] Geetha K, Dhanalakshmi A, Judie A. A study to assess the impact of leprosy on quality of life among leprosy patients in government rehabilitation home at Paranur. International Journal of Pharmaceutical and Clinical Research. 2015;7(6):466-468

[9] World Health Organization. Regional Office for the Western Pacific. Epidemiological Review of Leprosy in the WHO Western Pacific Region 2000. Manila: WHO/WPR; 2002. Available from: https://apps.who.int/iris/handle/10665/207775

[10] Pirayyavaraporn C, Peerapakorn S. The epidemiological impact of multidrug therapy. Leprosy Review. 1996;**67**:18-27

[11] Mgint T, Htoon MT. Leprosy in Myanmar, epidemiology and operational changes 1958-1992. Leprosy Review. 1996;**67**:18-27

[12] Jakeman P, Jakeman NRP, Singay J. Trends in leprosy in the Kingdom of Bhutan, 1982-1992. Leprosy Review. 1995;**66**:69-75

[13] Khang TH, Thanh LT, Lanh PH. Predictive value of gelatin particle agglutination test (GPAT) in leprosy detection. Indian Journal of Leprosy. 2018;**90**:61-67

[14] World Health Organization. Weekly Epidemiological Record. 2012;**34**:24

[15] Fajardo TT Jr, Villahermosa LG, Cruz EC, et al. A clinical trial of pefloxacin and ofloxacin in lepromatous leprosy. Leprosy Review. 2004;**75**(4):389-397

[16] Ji B et al. Ofloxacin for the treatment of leprosy. Acta Leprologica. 1991;7(4):321-326

[17] do Socorro Silva Costa P, Vianna FSL. Erythema nodosum leprosum: Update and challenge on the treatment of a neglected condition. Acta Tropica. 2018;**183**:134-141

[18] Han XY, Seo YH, Sizer KC, et al. A new *Mycobacterium* species causing diffuse Lepromatous leprosy. American Journal of Clinical Pathology. 2008;**130**:856-864

[19] Han XY, Silva FJ. On the age of leprosy. PLoS Neglected Tropical Diseases. 2014;**8**:e2544

[20] Bharadwaj VP, Katoch K. Detection of subclinical infection in leprosy: An 8 years follow up study. Indian Journal of Leprosy. 1989;**61**:495450

[21] Brett SJ, Draper P, Payne SN, et al. Serologic activity of a characteristic phenolic glycolipid from *Mycabacterium leprae* in sera from patients with leprosy and tuberculosis. Clinical and Experimental Immunology. 1983;**52**:271-279

[22] World Health Organization. Leprosy Elimination Projects: Status Report. Available from: https://apps.who.int/iris/handle/10665/68406

[23] Rao PN, Suneetha S, Pratap DV. Comparative study of uniform-MDT and WHO-MDT in Pauci and multi bacillary leprosy patients over 24 months of observation. Leprosy Review. 2009;**80**:143-155

[24] Kroger A, Pannikar V, Htoon MT, et al. International open trial of uniform multi-drug therapy regimen for 6 months for all types of leprosy patients: Rationale, design and preliminary results. Tropical Medicine & International Health. 2008;**13**:594-602

[25] Penna GO, Pontes MA, Cruz R, et al. Clinical trial for uniform multidrug therapy for leprosy patients in Brazil: Rationale and design. Memórias do Instituto Oswaldo Cruz. 2012;**107**:22-27

[26] Penna ML, Buhrer-Sekula S, Pontes MA, et al. Primary results of clinical trial of uniform multidrug therapy for leprosy patients in Brazil (U-MDT/CT-BR): Reactions frequency in multibacillary patients. Leprosy Review. 2012;**83**:308-319

[27] Penna ML, Buhrer-Sekula S, Pontes MA, et al. Results from the clinical trial of uniform multidrug therapy for leprosy patients in Brazil (U-MDT/CT-BR): Decrease in bacteriological index. Leprosy Review. 2014;**85**:262-266

[28] Ponder E, Moree M. Developing New Drugs & Vaccines for Neglected Diseases of the Poor. BIO Ventures for Global Health; 2012. p. 45

[29] Global Leprosy Strategy 2016-2020: Accelerating Towards a Leprosy-Free World. World Health Organization, Regional Office for South-East Asia: WHO; 2016

[30] Penna GO, Bührer-Sékula S, Ker LRS, et al. Uniform multidrug therapy for leprosy patients in Brazil (U-MDT/CT-BR): Final results of open label, randomized and controlled clinical trial, among MB patients. PLoS Neglected Tropical Diseases. 2017;**11**:e0005725

Chapter 7

Impact of Reconstructive Surgery (RCS) among Leprosy Patients: A Social Appraisal

Debajanee Lenka, Amarendra Mohapatra and Chittaranjan Kar

Abstract

Reconstructive surgery (RCS) has made a significant improvement in deformities and disabilities management among leprosy patients. However, it seems that due to existing misconceptions that is hereditary and not curable regarding leprosy still lead to concealing the disease, therefore the patients hesitate and unenthusiastic to avail these facilities. This study was carried out in Sonepur district of Odisha with 60 RCS has undertaken leprosy patients. Out of 71 operative patients during 2000–2012, only 60 patients were alive and interviewed, in this study entire universe was used without any sampling. A semi-structured questionnaire was administered to assess their understanding, better quality of life (QOL) after reconstructive surgery. Nearly, 98.6% could meet their expectations to some extent, another 1.6% failed to get their expectations. Among all the RCS patients only 33.3% changed their profession to avoid further risk in their life after surgery. This study concludes that Reconstructive surgery plays a vital role to bring for leprosy patients into their normal life and lead their life in this open society of today. The result implies a motivational message for the deformed leprosy patients to come forward and depicts to encourage the surgeons to counsel the patients towards reconstructive surgery, which will reduce stigma in due course.

Keywords: leprosy, stigma, RCS, QOL, knowledge, acceptance

1. Introduction

Leprosy is a chronic infectious disease caused by *Mycobacterium leprae* (*M. leprae*). It is a micro-organism which has a predilection for soft tissues of a human organism like skin and nerve. Now leprosy is known as a common cause of non-traumatic peripheral neuropathy worldwide [1]. This *Mycobacterium leprae*, the causative agent of leprosy, was first discovered by Hansen in 1873. Therefore leprosy is also known as Hansen's disease and considering it the first bacterium to be identified as causing disease in human [2].

The transmission of *Mycobacterium leprae* always occurs through upper airways and manifested as skin lesions with reducing sensation including nodule, pigmentation, and patches on some portion of the body. These lesions can affect any part of the body as a nasal bridge and oral cavity [3]. The above said causative agent of leprosy, *Mycobacterium bacillus*, is associated with a prolonged incubation period between initial infection and development of skin reactions. The incubation period of leprosy is 5–10 years but it hardly takes 20 years to have appeared as skin patches, deformities, and disabilities [4].

The extent of social stigma aggravates due to the blind believe or the misconception that leprosy is not curable and is hereditary. The crippled limbs (finger and feet) add fuel to fire of social stigma.

Reconstructive surgery to correct deformities in leprosy has made dramatic and revolutionary changes in the lives of affected patients [5, 6]. Nevertheless, leprosy patients are still hesitating to avail these benefits of reconstructive surgery due to many reasons [7]. The existing reasons associated with leprosy lead to take delay treatment and concealment of disease in society.

Since history, the misconceptions about leprosy being a hereditary disease, lead to increase the level of stigma related to death and mutilation due to its existing attributed causes like deformity and disability. This misconception also leads to prejudice, discrimination and social exclusion which are resulting in infliction of congenital suffering on leprosy patients, which can have serious repercussions in their personal and professional lives [8].

Government integrated Reconstructive surgery unit in the health care system to reduce stigma, which caused due to misconceptions, and to eliminate leprosy burden in different states of our country with the help of PPP (Public-private partnership) program including Government and non-government organizations Contemporary to Govt. The non-government organization has put more efforts. NGOs had handled 1076 surgery cases whereas Government hospitals had done 921. Maharastra has performed a better result in comparison to other states with 495 RCS by both Government and NGO. The recorded data on Reconstructive surgery has been given below (**Table 1**).

Table 1 shows that among 35 states all across India, Maharastra has performed well at both Government and NGO level, i.e., 39 and 456. Next to Andhra Pradesh NGO has performed 487 RCS. In Madhya Pradesh, the government has done 122, whereas 91 was performed by NGO. Similarly, Odisha has performed very nicely in Government level, i.e., 248 RCS in 2013–2014 and Chhattisgarh has performed as well in same Government level with 234 RCS than 5 in NGO. In NGO level the performance of RCS is far better than Government. In Uttar Pradesh, 235 RCS has carried out in NGO and 33 in Govt level. But some states have not performed satisfactorily in both. Thus, it gives an idea of RCS (1786) has been well performed in NGO level.

1.1 State

The present research has been conducted in Odisha, consists of 30 districts. Among these districts, seven designated surgical units have been inaugurated in few districts for leprosy RCS. These districts are Berhampur, Dhenkanal, Koraput, Sonepur, and Cuttack, etc. In Odisha 10 government institution and 5 NGOs have been recognized for performing RCS. In Odisha, the number of Reconstructive Surgery performed by the Government is 262 in 2012–2013, 248 in 2013–2014 and 307 in 2014–2015 (end of March) whereas NGO has not performed any RCS.

Figure 1 the NGO-LEPRA Institutional Based Rehabilitation (IBR) is working tirelessly on post rehabilitation of RCS patients and provides free footwear and skill development training. The health staffs of this IBR have taken endeavour to aware the people about the system for early diagnosis and available Government facilities for leper patients.

In Odisha many studies have been conducted on leprosy, its stigma and how does it affect man and women, its community perception and knowledge about its

Sl. no	State	Inst. recognized for RCS		RCS performed	
		Govt.	NGO	Govt.	NGO
1	Andhra Pradesh	1	9	0	487
2	Arunachal Pradesh	0	0	0	0
3	Assam	1	1	0	16
4	Bihar	2	2	21	64
5	Chhattisgarh	1	2	234	5
6	Goa	1	0	0	0
7	Gujrat	3	0	136	0
8	Haryana	1	0	0	0
9	Himachal Pradesh	0	0	0	0
10	Jharkhand	2	3	10	47
11	Jammu & Kashmir	0	0	0	0
12	Karnataka	5	4	34	106
13	Kerala	0	2	0	0
14	Madhya Pradesh	2	1	122	91
15	Maharastra	9	8	39	456
16	Manipur	1	0	0	0
17	Meghalaya	0	0	0	0
18	Mizoram	0	0	0	0
19	Nagaland	0	0	0	0
20	Odisha	10	5	248	0
21	Punjab	0	0	0	0
22	Rajasthan	1	0	2	0
23	Sikkim	1	0	1	0
24	Tamilnadu	2	8	1	106
25	Tripura	0	0	0	0
26	Uttar Pradesh	3	2	33	235
27	Uttarakhand	1	0	15	0
28	West Bengal	9	2	18	90
29	A&N Island	0	0	0	0
30	Chandigarh	1	0	0	0
31	D&N Haveli	0	0	0	0
32	Daman and Diu	0	0	0	0
33	Delhi	2	2	5	83
34	Lakshadweep	0	0	0	0
35	Pondicherry	1	0	2	0
Total		60	51	921	1786

No. of RCS performed in different states of India 2013–2014 (NLEP progress report on 2013–2014, dt.26/8/2015) [9].

Table 1.
Institutes and No. of RCS cases operated state wise.

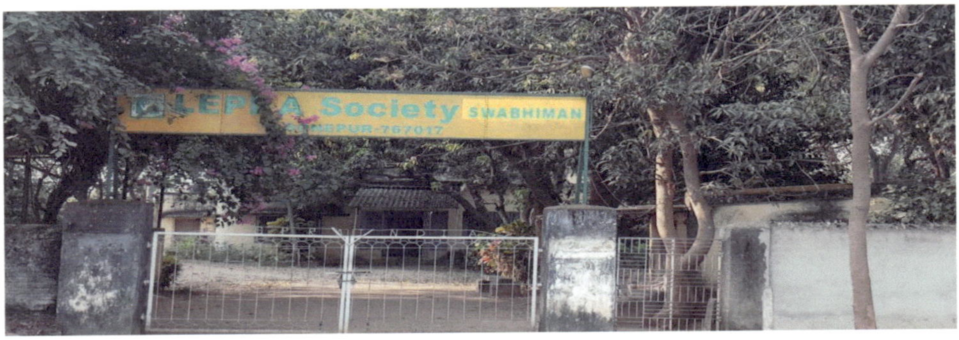

Figure 1.
An IBR of lepers at Sonepur.

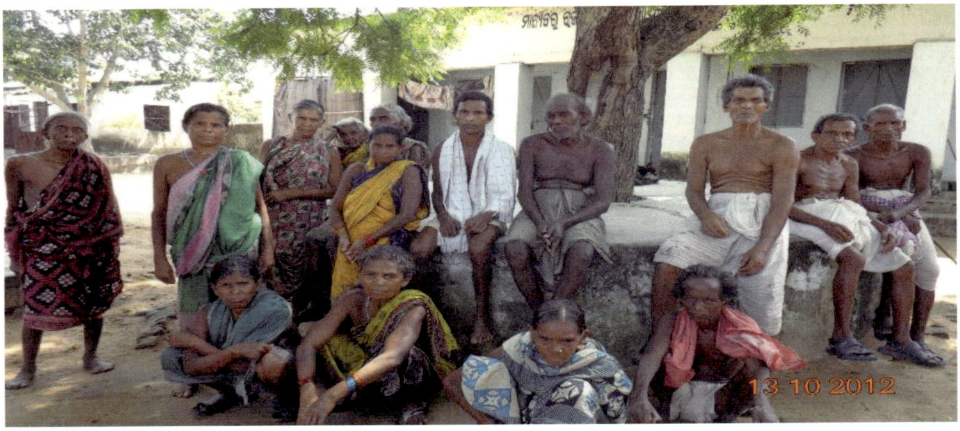

Figure 2.
Lepers at Kustha ashram.

treatment, etc. But no literature is available on patients' perception after surgery. So the intention of this work is to explore the patients' perception regarding post RCS and its consequences. This study is conducted in Sonepur district of Odisha; the LEPRA society office at Sonepur has a rehabilitation center for leprosy patients. They did help me in getting the old patients contacts.

The aim of this study is to assess the patients' socio-psychological condition and their acceptance in society after reconstructive surgery.

Figure 2 depicts about the lepers of Kustha Ashram in Sonepur district, Odisha. It has been established in the year 2001 by the Government to facilitate the isolated deformed and disability lepers from society. Government supports the patients to rehabilitate them by supplying footwear, cloth, food along with pay pension, widow pension and compensation for surgery who have undergone for RCS.

2. Methodology

The study area was selected according to the highest prevalence and annual case detection rate of leprosy in Odisha. In the year 2009–2010, the highest ANCDR was 41.7% of Sonepur district in comparison to another endemic zone of Odisha. During this study, the record of surgery patients reported that 71 had undergone for surgery of six different blocks of Sonepur district. Out of these RCS patients list, only 60 RCS patients were alive and included in this study, which is the universe sample of this study area. In this work above age 60+ and below 15 year leprosy patients, non-RCS patients in leprosy were excluded. This study was conducted in three phases like pilot study, main field work-1, and main fieldwork-2.

In Pilot study, which was conducted for 4 weeks to interact with patients, health staffs like MO, DLO and Paramedical health staffs who were working in leprosy. A semi-structured questionnaire was developed and examined various tools for the assessment of RCS patients. In the first phase of the main fieldwork, data pertaining to the demographic profile of the patients and their household and the quality of life were gathered from reconstructive surgery leprosy patients.

In the second phase of the main fieldwork, data pertaining to social and psychological consequences were gathered from leprosy patients and interaction with their caregivers and family members is carried out. Then a number of case studies with leprosy patients, two rounds of focus group discussion (FGD) with different stakeholders such as, patients, family members, and health staff were collected from all six blocks of Sonepur district which were hectic.

Limitation of this study was following the subject participants at their place of residence or was a daunting task as they were dispersed in the wide area of six blocks. To some extent, it became a limitation due to inadequate time and inconvenient traveling to communicate the patients, their respective family members and the varied socio-cultural set-ups where they are living.

3. Result

3.1 Patients selection

All the Reconstructive surgery patients of Sonepur district were selected for the purpose of this study. It was reported that 71 patients had surgery but only 60 could be interviewed and others were migrated/died. All the patients were dispersed in six blocks of this above-said district.

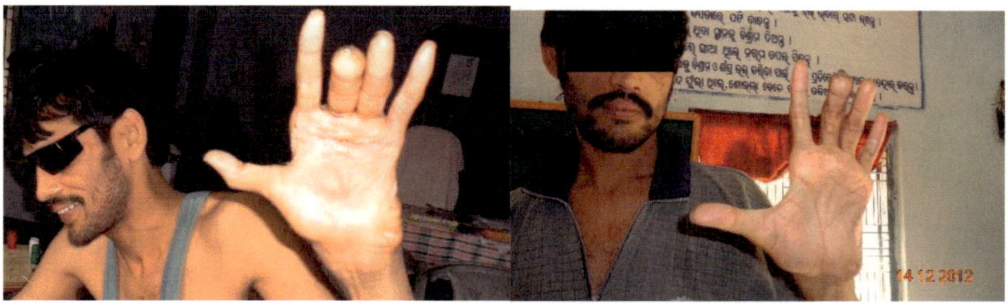

Pre RCS

Post RCS

Table 2 represents the effect of RCS among the undergone surgery patients. Deformities were observed in both hand and feet of the registered RCS patients. Before surgery, 48.3% had deformities in their hands and needed full assistance but after surgery, only 18.3% required help from others. Out of 60 RCS patients, 54% had hand deformities but some extent they could manage their work. In the third parameter, after surgery, 96.6% did not need the assistance of anyone. Similarly, in feet deformities only 10% required full assistance after surgery and 93.3% need no assistance. This above table reveals that RCS enables a patient to perform all activities of hand and feet independently.

Deformities occurred body organ	Parameters	Before (%)	After (%)
Hand	Full assistance	29 (48.3)	11 (18.3)
	Some assistance	54 (90)	18 (30)
	No assistance	20 (33.3)	58 (96.6)
Feet	Full assistance	12 (20)	06 (10)
	Some assistance	19 (31.6)	04 (6.6)
	No assistance	54 (90)	56 (93.3)

Table 2.
Quality of life of pre and post RCS patients.

Table 3 elaborates on the satisfaction of the patients with society as a whole pre RCS. It gives data about the satisfaction level obtained from family members, friends, relatives, society and their over-all life.

In the case of the family, none of the patients are very satisfied with the acceptance of their family members. Out of 60 patients, 54, i.e., 90%, were partially satisfied with the behavior and acceptance of their family members in pre RCS. Six patients, i.e., 10%, were dissatisfied with their family members pre RCS.

In the case of friends only one, i.e., 1.6% patient found to be very satisfied with the acceptance of his friend before RCS. Forty-nine patients, i.e., 81.6% were partially satisfied by the acceptance of friends. Ten patients, i.e., 16.6% were fully dissatisfied by the behavior of their friends pre RCS.

Only one patient (1.6%) is fully satisfied with the acceptance of relatives before RCS. Eighty percent, i.e., 48 patients out of 60 were partially satisfied with the relatives before RCS, 11 patients, i.e., 18.3% were fully dissatisfied with the behavior of the relatives with them pre RCS.

If we take society as a whole, only one patient, i.e., 1.6% was fully satisfied with the society pre RCS stage. Forty-two patients, i.e., 70% were partially satisfied with the society before RCS. Seventeen patients, i.e., 28.3% were fully dissatisfied with the society before RCS.

The disease is such that no one can be satisfied with overall life. Only one patient, i.e., 1.6% was in spite of the disease fully satisfied with his overall life. Sixteen patients, i.e., 26.6% are partially satisfied with overall life. Forty-three patients, i.e., 71.6% are fully dissatisfied with their overall life.

Sl. no	Parameters	Very satisfied (%)	Partially satisfied (%)	Dissatisfied (%)
Pre RCS				
1	How satisfied are you with your acceptance by family	0 (0)	54 (90)	6 (10)
2	How satisfied are you with your acceptance by friends	1 (1.60)	49(81.60)	10 (16.6)
3	How satisfied are you with your acceptance by relatives	1 (1.60)	48 (80)	11 (18.3)
4	How satisfied are you with your acceptance by society	1 (1.60)	42 (70)	17 (28.3)
5	How satisfied about your overall life	1 (1.60)	16 (26.6)	43 (71.6)

Table 3.
Quality of social relation and support of pre RCS patients.

Table 4 presents the result of Post RCS acceptance and support. Almost 86% of patients are very satisfied with the acceptance of their family, friend, relatives, and society. But 47 (78.3%) patients showed their satisfaction on overall life. After surgery among all the criteria of acceptance, 20% replied they are partially satisfied upon their life which is greater than other cases. In other cases, only 11–13% of patients answered they feel less satisfied. A very negligible percentage of patients have been counted in the dissatisfy column. Thus, **Table 4** shows better result and improvement in the patient's life after reconstructive surgery when compared to **Table 3**.

Table 5 and **Figure 3** depict that after surgery among the 60 reconstructive surgery patients only 20 (33.3%) patients had changed their profession as they still had little loss of sensation in hand and feet and so they preferred a profession which needed less movement and it was flexible for them to adopt. After surgery patients were suggested to take rest for 6 months and go to work only after complete healing. So only 40 patients could prefer their same old profession presently people believe that absence of deformity is the only concern of society for an individual to lead his/her life as a normal being. Many research work on leprosy stated that deformity is creating a social stigma against this disease in society. So after surgery, it is proved that "no deformity is equal to no stigma." RCS has given a great effort to reduce the pressure of social stigma from society.

3.2 Economic status

Figure 4 describes the economic status of the patients after and before the RCS. Before RCS 35% of patients' income was below Rs. 1000 but however, in post RCS it is found that only 21.6% of patients income was below Rs. 1000. Similarly, the income of 60% was between Rs. 1000 and 5000 in Pre RCS but it increased to 66.6% in post RCS. 8.3% of patients' had earned Rs. 6000–10,000 which was only 5% in patients before surgery. In post RCS only 3.3% patient could get above Rs. 10,000 but in Pre-surgery, no one was capable to earn this much amount. So it is concluded that RCS has helped the patients to earn more than what they earned before RCS and the economic status of the patients has improved to a great level. The highest number of patients are earning a minimum amount between Rs. 1000 and 5000 because most of the patients belong to the farming profession.

Sl. no.	Parameters	Very satisfied (%)	Partially satisfied (%)	Dissatisfied (%)
Post RCS				
1	How satisfied are you with your acceptance by family	51 (85)	8 (13.30)	1 (1.60)
2	How satisfied are you with your acceptance by friends	52 (86.60)	6 (10)	2 (3.30)
3	How satisfied are you with your acceptance by relatives	52 (86.60)	6 (10)	2 (3.30)
4	How satisfied are you with your acceptance by society	51 (85)	7 (11.60)	2 (3.30)
5	How satisfied about your overall life	47 (78.30)	12 (20)	1 (1.60)

Table 4.
Impact of RCS on social relationship and support of post RCS patients.

Serial number	Change in occupation	Number of patients (%)
1	Farming	6 (10)
2	Business	3 (5)
3	Job	4 (6.6)
4	Others	7 (11.7)
Total		20 (33.3)

Table 5.
Incidence of RCS patients changing profession.

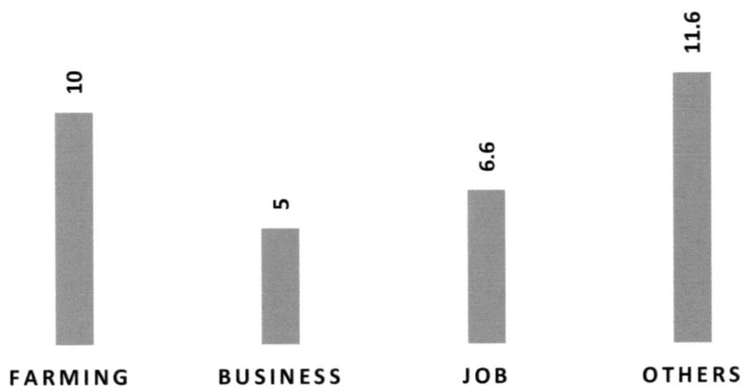

Figure 3.
Changed profession in post RCS.

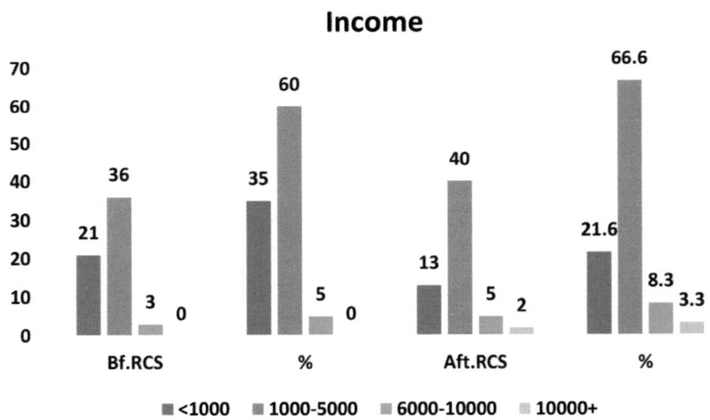

Figure 4.
Economic profile.

4. Discussion

The purpose of the study is to assess the quality of life for those who had undergone RCS with leprosy. The overall result shows that after reconstructive surgery performance of patients have improved due to better mobility of limbs. 96.6% reported that they do not need others to support to meet their expectations. This result is comparable with the similar study of John in which he explained more than 50% patients said that after correction of deformities they could meet their expectations [10], subjectively assessed, 85% and above were satisfied with their social acceptance with respect to family, relatives, and peers, 13% were partially satisfied and 2% were dissatisfied. These results were corroborating with that of Ebenezer et al.'s study [11]. Similarly, Virmond and Palande stated that RCS has undergone patients' income and acceptance which was reduced to a great extent before disease, again regained. Therefore, they opined that early correction of disabilities prevents dehabilitation [12]. When it was discussed in regard to depression and anxiety of leprosy patients, a psychological study of Ramanathan et al. explained that 25 randomly selected patients undergoing corrective surgical procedure for their disabilities and deformities, high anxiety and depression levels were found preoperatively and in contrast to the result of the present study only 40% could meet their expectations [13]. After interaction with all the RCS patients, it was observed that they followed the doctor's advice for 6 months complete rest and avoided to lift heavy materials. This had helped them for complete recovery and no complications for which the satisfaction level is high 85%. If we discuss about the gender difference in the impact of leprosy; women with leprosy are more vulnerable than men in respect to all aspects like relationship, acceptance and workability. This study observed that 6.6% women were separated, rejected and avoided by their family and community members. These similar findings were observed in Mull et al. study which was conducted in Karachi. They reported that the proportion of diagnosed male with leprosy were high than female. They observed that women were not forewarned about MDT regimens and it might have been due to practice of purdah and lack of female health worker [14]. In addition, Naik et al. explained that women faced more domestic violence and deprived from personal contacts with others [15]. Similarly, Carol et al. and Janna et al. reported that women are more vulnerable because they were derived from personal contact with their family as well as community. Even they observed that women were more sufferers from rejection and isolation [16, 17]. Besides, according to psychological domain, Oliveira and Romanelli reported that female leprosy patients tend to neglected themselves, that the fear of abandonment, stigma and they are concerned about their appearance [18]. In addition Mankar et al. measured the QOL for the sexes and found it relatively higher impact of leprosy on women than the control leprosy patients [19]. Thus deformity and disabilities among patients made them to deprive from work activities. Another study of Natasja et al. explained that comparison of SLASA scale assessment on limitation of activities of the patients after 1 year it revealed that those had reconstructive surgery showed a significant improvement in their activities but there was no significant change found among them who declined RCS. Thus, concluded that reconstructive surgery has a beneficial effect on the functioning of limbs [20]. This present study result showed that due to the avoidance of further difficulties in their life only 33% changed their profession. It was earlier stated by Dharmendra that, "the beggar problem is a difficult one in India as the money and institutions needed for them are not available" [21]. Thus, it has been reported that in many studies: begging is the ideal profession of leprosy patients. One of these papers of Harvinder and Brakel, they specified that isolation and prohibition of the patients make them incapable to do any profession for their livelihood. Therefore, they choose to beg as their profession and stick to it till the end of their life [22]. If we consider the income of surgery patients before RCS they faced problem due to their deformities and lost strength to continue their work. Thus their socioeconomic status is categorized as per SES scale of Kuppuswamy into five groups. Sixty percent were earning Rs. 1000–5000 and no one was getting 10,000. After surgery 3.3% are earning more than 10,000 and <5 people were in <1000 and rest was in the bracket of Rs. 6000–10,000 with SES scale. This suggests that RCS brought an economic upliftment, which gave them social status and security. ($ = 70.30/– and £ = 90.39).

5. Conclusion

Reconstructive surgery (RCS) had revealed the visible impact among the leprosy patients. This study concludes that patients who had undergone RCS have improved quality of life when compare to their past experience before RCS and with those who are still concealing the deformities and disabilities without availing the RCS facilities due to social stigma. It may be noted that in case of leprosy the self-stigma dominates among all leprosy patients. This needs a proper counseling at family level to understand the disease, its curability nature and that is not a hereditary by nature. This study reports that post RCS acceptance by society and the level of quality of overall life has improved to 78.3% from 1.6% in pre-surgery. Similarly, the performance of limbs in post RCS is very satisfactory, i.e., 96.6% in hand and 93.3% in foot mobility.

The findings of this present work will hopefully could motivate the hidden and concealed cases to come forward and avail the free surgery RCS in designated centers. In turn, the surgeons would also be encouraged for their great effort which could reduce social stigma among these leprosy patients. It will also help to dispel the misconception about disease and create awareness about diagnosis and treatment. Thus, RCS reduces the social stigma in a significant way.

Acknowledgements

The authors gratefully acknowledge the LEPRA society, District Leprosy Officer (DLO) and Para Medical staffs who facilitated the research, RCS leprosy patients who shared their stories, my co-workers and the interpreter Manoj Bhoi.

Conflict of interest

The authors declare that there is no conflict of interest regarding the publication of this chapter.

Abbreviations

RCS	reconstructive surgery
QOL	quality of life
ANCDR	annual case detection rate
PPP	public private partnership
NGO	non-government organization
M. leprae	*Mycobacterium leprae*
NLEP	National Leprosy Elimination Programme
DLO	District Leprosy Officer
MO	Medical Officer

Author details

Debajanee Lenka[1,2]*, Amarendra Mohapatra[2] and Chittaranjan Kar[3]

1 Department of Anthropology, Utkal University, Bhubaneswar, Odisha, India

2 ICMR-Regional Medical Research Centre, Bhubaneswar Dist-Khurda, Odisha, India

3 Department of Nephrology, SCB Medical College and Hospital, Cuttack, Odisha, India

*Address all correspondence to: r.debajanee@gmail.com

References

[1] Ramachandra AG. Reconstructive surgery as preparation for rehabilitation. Leprosy in India. 1969;**41**:210-211

[2] Srinivas H. "Prevention of Disabilities in Patients with Leprosy": A Practical Guide. Geneva: World Health Organization; 1963

[3] Dawn AG, Lee PP. Patients expectations for medical and surgical care: A review of the literature and applications to ophthalmology. Survey of Ophthalmology. 2004;**49**:513-524

[4] Araujo MG. Hansen no Brasil. Revista da Sociedade Brasileira de Medicina Tropical. 2003;**36**:373-382

[5] GHA H. Investigations concerning the etiology of leprosy. Norsk Magazin for Lagevidenkaben. 1874;**4**:1-88

[6] Mareno CMC, Enders BC, Simpson CA. Evaluation of leprosy skills: Opinion of doctors and nurses of family health teams. Revista Brasileira de Enfermagem. 2008;**61**(Br):671-675

[7] Ministry of Health, Secretariat of Health Surveillance. Department of Epidemiological Surveillance. Health Surveillance: Epidemiological Situation of Leprosy in Brazil. Brazil: Ministry of Health; 2008

[8] Baialadri KS. The stigma of leprosy: Report of a group experience with people with HIV. Hansenologia Internationalis. 2007;**32**:27-36

[9] NLEP Progress Report on 2013-2014. Available from: www.nlep.org.in

[10] Annamma S, John D, Kumar V, Rao PSS. Patient's perceptions of reconstructive surgery in leprosy. Leprosy Review. 2005;**76**:48-54

[11] Ebenezer M, Rao K, Partheebaranjan S. Factors affecting functional outcome of surgical correction of claw hand in leprosy. Indian Journal of Leprosy. 2012;**84**:259-264

[12] Palande DD, Marcos V. Social rehabilitation and surgery in leprosy. Hansenologia Internationalis. 2002;**27**(2):99-104

[13] Ramanathan U, Malaviya GN, Jain N, Husain S. Psycholosocial aspects of deformed leprosy patients undergoing surgical correction. Leprosy Review. 1991;**62**:402-409

[14] Mull JD et al. Culture and compliance among leprosy patients in Pakistan. Social Science and Medicine. 1989;**29**(7):799-811

[15] Naik SS et al. Problems and needs of women leprosy patients in Bombay and Goa—A preliminary report. Indian Journal of Leprosy. 1991;**63**(2):213-222

[16] Carol V et al. Double jeopardy: Women and leprosy in India. World Health Statistics Quarterly. Rapport Trimestriel de Statistiques Sanitaires Mondiales. 1996;**49**:120-126

[17] Dijkstra Janna IR, Van Brakel WH, Van Elteren M. Gender and leprosy related stigma in endemic areas: A systematic review. Leprosy Review. 2017;**88**:419-440

[18] Romaneilli O. The effects of leprosy on men and women: A gender study. Cadernos de Saúde Pública. 1998;**14**:51-60

[19] Mankar MJ, Joshi SM, Velankar DH, et al. A comparative study of the quality of life, knowledge, attitude and belief about leprosy disease among leprosy patients and community members in shantivan leprosy—Rehabilitation center, Nere, Maharastra, India. Journal of Global Infectious Diseases. 2011;**3**:378-382

[20] Van veen Natasja HJ, Hemo Dinabandhu A, Bowers Robert L, David P, et al. Evaluation of activity limitation and social participation, and effects of reconstructive surgery in people with disability due to leprosy: A prospective cohort study. Disability and Rehabilitation. 2011;**33**(8):667-674

[21] Dharmendra. Social aspects of leprosy. Leprosy in India. 1954;**26**:113-120

[22] Harvinder K, Van Wim B. Is beggary a chosen profession among people living in a leprosy colony. Leprosy Review. 2002;**73**:334-345

Chapter 8

Neglected Tropical Diseases Pathogen and Human Genetic Interaction in the Genomic Era: Opportunities for (Sub-Saharan) African Scientists to Get on Board

Issiaka Soulama

Abstract

The worldwide prevalence of the neglected tropical diseases (NTD) shows the diseases are affecting more than 1 billion. The burden of the Neglected tropical diseases cost to developing, the burden of the diseases cost to developing economies billions of dollars every year. The genomic research in the last decades providing a full sequence (some currently in the sequencing pipeline) of genomes of many of the organisms including those which are responsible of neglected tropical diseases, may help in the management of such diseases. With the human genome being sequenced, the understanding of the genomic interaction between human and NTD pathogen enable scientists to develop new strategies to prevent and treat these devastating diseases. In this context of genomic era, African scientists may interestingly play an insider role in order to be part of the history of the elimination of these diseases. However, a critical mass of African scientists in genomic area constitutes the first step toward this long way in struggle against NTD. Although the challenge is enormous, it is very important to recognize that some African countries and institutions are fully committed to develop and strengthen African leadership in genomic area, while some are conspicuously absent from this debate. Joining African competences and leadership through collaborative activities and moving forward remains the next challenge to really impact the control and elimination of the NTD.

Keywords: NTD, genomic, scientists, elimination, Africa

1. Introduction

The neglected tropical diseases (NTDs) are known as a group of bacterial, parasitic, viral, and fungal infections strongly associated with poverty with an increase overlapping in tropical areas. They occurred particularly in areas affected by socioeconomic progress and unfortunately combined with other factors such as limited access to safe water and sanitation, chronic hunger, and also in areas where vector-transmitted diseases are more frequent. According to the World Bank Study, Sub-Saharan Africa population represents the major focus for the NTDs [1] and as mentioned from the 2010 Global Burden of Disease Study, NTDs accounted for more than 26 million [2]. Most of the NTDs are well known as ancient diseases resulting in humanity concerns for centuries [3]. From the 2020 Roadmap, 20 NTDs were identified as following: Buruli ulcer, Chagas disease, cysticercosis/taeniasis, dengue fever, dracunculiasis (guinea worm disease), echinococcosis, food-borne trematodiasis, human African trypanosomiasis (HAT) (sleeping sickness), leishmaniasis, leprosy, lymphatic filariasis, onchocerciasis (river blindness), rabies, schistosomiasis, soil-transmitted helminthiasis (ascariasis, hookworm, and trichuriasis), trachoma, and yaws [4]. The World Health Organization classified the NTDs into two mains groups: in one hand the preventive chemotherapy and transmission control (PCT) NTDs including prominently lymphatic filariasis, onchocerciasis, schistosomiasis, and soil-transmitted helminthiasis while the innovative and intensified disease management (IDM) on the other hand is constitute with Buruli ulcer, Chagas disease, human African trypanosomiasis, and leishmaniasis disease that are currently lack suitable tools for large scale use [5]. NTDs remain as a public health problem for poor populations living in tropical environments and difficult-to-access areas with more than 40% of impacted people living in the WHO African Region. The challenge is as much as important to justify the development of a specific program at WHO AFRO which mission is to provide technical orientation, support and guidance to Member States in the WHO African region. The development of genomic represents an opportunity that can contribute to the accelerated prevention, control, elimination, and eradication of NTDs and neglected zoonoses.

2. Geographical distribution and global burden of the NTDs

The concept, the burden, and the geographical repartition of the NTDs (**Figure 1**) justify the need of a global advocacy including the health policy-makers and ultimately the opportunity for tackling the NTDs with the same urgency and the commitment as for HIV/AIDS, tuberculosis, and malaria [6].

As previously well described by Hotez [6–8], the NTDs are characterized by the following important elements:

- Described as the most common infections of people living in sub-Saharan Africa, Asia, and Latin America and the Caribbean where the poverty is known as the component.

- NTDs affect about 1.4 billion people who live below the World Bank poverty figure of US$1.25 per day.

- Unfortunately, the NTDs result in chronic infections lasting years or even decades resulting in a great impact on the affected people family revenue.

- The chronicity of The NTDs affect child growth and intellectual and cognitive developments, impair pregnancy outcomes, and decrease worker productivity and then the billions of affected people cannot escape poverty.

- Among the consequence, the NTDs also cause blindness and disfigurement that are psychologically devastating and result in social stigma.

- This high level of morbidity, economic impairment, and stigma does not necessarily translate into large numbers of deaths; overall, the NTDs cause high-morbidity but low-mortality conditions.

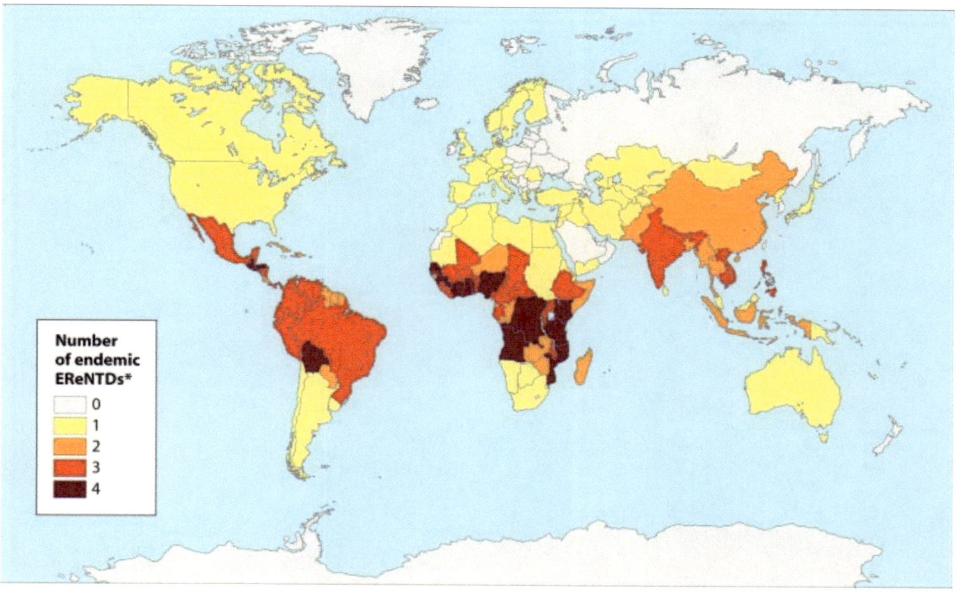

Figure 1.
Global intensity map of EReNTD regions of endemicity. Data are from the World Health Organization (2013).

Regarding the chronicity of the disease but also as diseases afflicting humankind for centuries, NTDs are considered as "non-emerging" disease in contrast to emerging infections such as HIV/AIDS, SARS, and avian influenza.

Moreover, based on the previous studies, it is well documented that there is a geographic overlap among seven of the NTDs (ascariasis, trichuriasis, hookworm infection, schistosomiasis, LF, onchocerciasis, and trachoma). This is especially observed in sub-Saharan Africa where those NTDs present a very high prevalence. However, the overlapping of the NTDs in this part of the world allow to target these conditions simultaneously by combining the drugs in an integrated concept so named "rapid-impact package" [7, 9], as the drugs can be easily and quickly deployed by a contingent of community drug distributors. The rapid-impact package strategy if well implemented should ultimately contribute to the interruption of the diseases transmission such LF, onchocerciasis, and trachoma [9].

3. Impact of NTDs on public health

Although the NTDs are known to severely impact everyone, the diseases affect women and girls disproportionately for the following reasons:

Biological and physiological factors of *women and girls* lead to increased vulnerability of this specific category to particular pathologies—for example, female genital schistosomiasis and severe helminth-related anemia in pregnant women.

Socio-cultural factors are suspected in increasing risk to NTDs. A specific notified example is the water-based domestic activities carried out in two-third Sub-Saharan Africa by women or girls which increases risk of diseases such as schistosomiasis, whereas child-care and caregiving increases risk of trachoma and blindness. In fact, research suggested that women account for 80% of disability-adjusted life years linked to trachoma-related blindness.

NTDs that cause disfigurement and disability (such as lymphatic filariasis) can have a disproportionately negative impact on employability and marriageability

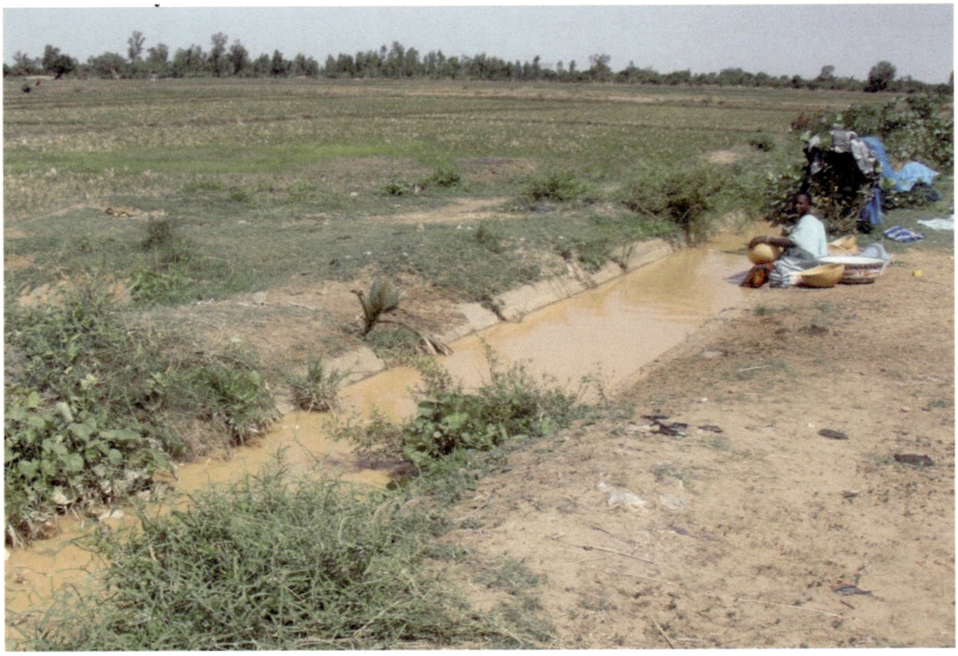

Figure 2.
A woman washing dishes in a canal. Image credit Anouk Gouvras.

of affected women, making them dependent on family members and potentially leading to stigmatization and social exclusion.

Indirect impact of NTDs can also disproportionately affect women and girls as caregivers, having to give up their jobs or drop out of school in order to take care of a sick family member (**Figure 2**).

4. Global mobilization and role of scientific commitment against neglected tropical disease

The worldwide burden of NTDs lead to a global mobilization with a development of a strategic work plan 2014–2020, which has been developed with the following objectives: scale up access to NTD-related interventions; enhance planning for results, resource mobilization, and financial sustainability of national NTD programs; strengthen advocacy, coordination, and national ownership; and enhance monitoring, evaluation, surveillance, and research [10] (WHO, 2012): Roadmap: accelerating work to overcome the global impact of neglected tropical diseases.

The 2020 roadmap against NTD recommend further research including the need for newer and safer drugs, vector control, personal hygiene, and the development of vaccines. In the implementation of the roadmap, there are several initiative including control programs or research initiatives bringing their resources and competences. Then, a more macro approach may be necessary to promote greater effectiveness in addressing the underlining social, human health, zoonotic, and environmental challenges to prevent morbidity, and mortality from these diseases. One such approach that is growing worldwide in recognition is the "One Health" initiative, a commitment of interdisciplinary and multistakeholder involved locally, nationally, and globally in areas of human and animal health, agriculture, and the environment [1–15]. However, these one health approaches should be sensitive to resource-poor settings and should leverage partners and broader global public health networks as it is represented in **Figure 3**.

Although there are many NGOs and partners committed in NTDs control, scientific commitment is quite negligible in designing strategies and implementation. However, very few of them are from Africa where most of the NTD are present. Although African scientist's mobilization and commitment are well practical in some of the NTD control, very few inputs is observed in the genetic and genomic area. Indeed, the control and the elimination of certain NTD will be rapidly and successfully carried out with the contribution of the understanding of human and pathogen genomic interaction. Interestingly genomic constitute the new insight generating from genetic studies that can provide explanations and may even allow predictions to be made, in the context of a range of biological problems including the field of inherited human disorders. The development of the genetic in the last decade leads ineluctably to the "genomic" era. Then, importantly, with the improvement of sequencing technologies and the enormous reduction in the cost of sequencing, biologists are facing with a "data avalanche." The development of the next generation whole exome or genome sequencing may bring to the scientific community large possibility of tools to elucidate genetic perturbation occurring in many diseases including the neglected tropical diseases. Consequently, genomic data analysis may also be useful for the dissection of the genetic mechanisms underlying complex polygenic diseases or in understanding how some modifiers genes can influence the age of onset or clinical severity of a given disease

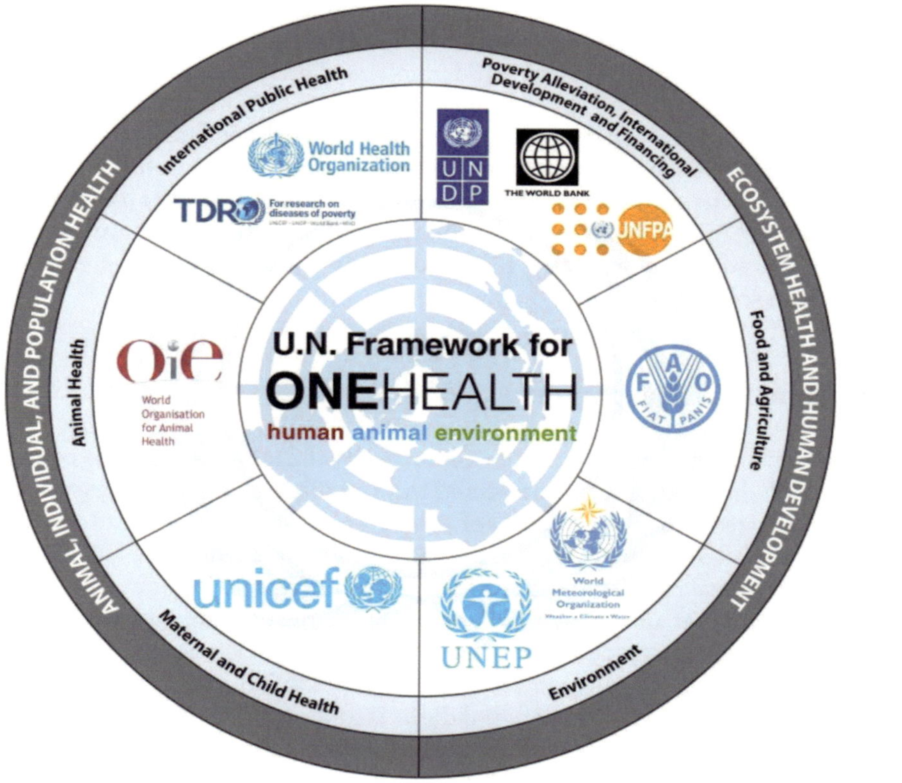

Figure 3.
Proposed United Nations "One Health" framework. FAO, Food and Agriculture Organization; OIE, World Organization for Animal Health; TDR, WHO Special Programme for Research and Training in Tropical Diseases; UNDP, United Nations Development Programme; UNEP, United Nations Environment Programme; UNFPA, United Nations Population Fund; UNICEP, United Nations Children's Fund; WHO, World Health Organization; WMO, World Meteorological Organization.

entity. Interestingly, while we are acquiring new research capabilities, we are also encountering new problems with the analysis of genomic data such as genomic data presentation, format, sharing, and reanalysis.

5. Programs and strategies ongoing in the field of genomic supporting the eradication of neglected tropical disease

The number of emerging infectious diseases is increasing annually despite the numerous of effort going on. In parallel to the wide incidence of the infectious disease including neglected tropical disease, characterizing novel or re-emerging infections is aided by the availability of pathogen genomes. This also helps to develop new approaches. Indeed, recently an *in silico* approach for discovering new filarial drug targets was developed in which comparative sequence analysis and functional genomics data from the related model nematode *Caenorhabditis elegans* are combined into subtractive filters that can be used to identify potentially essential nematode genes and generate a pool of pre-validated candidate targets [15–17]. Different techniques such as the RNA interference (RNAi) experiments and other functional studies serve as potential genomic tools to examine gene function from NTDs pathogen. Interestingly, sequencing of pathogen genomes, can contribute to describing nearly every aspect of transmission dynamics when some of the following information, date, location, clinical manifestation, or others data regarding the samples origin are including. The analyses of these data can positively affect the clinical management of the disease or the public health practice such as policies for surveillance, prevention, and treatment. The combination of genomic and epidemiological data represents consequently a perfect tool to address answers to epidemiological questions and reduce incidence and prevalence. How can genomic approaches support neglected tropical disease eradication particularly by analogy with how conservation genomics is supporting efforts to prevent extinctions. They are genomic approaches of capacity building programs in Africa as described through the next paragraphs that are contributing to reach this goal demonstrating the opportunity behind this cutting-edge method for African scientists.

6. Genomic training programs in Africa

Genomics remain one excellent component in the long way of NTD control and elimination. In order to tackle neglected tropical disease and move forward with elimination steps, the development of competent resources constitute one of the important challenge particularly in Sub-Saharan Africa, where the NTD present the highest prevalence. There are few institute in Africa taking the opportunity of genomic era that are focused and committed to the development of scientists with excellent competence and capacity in genomic. The global effort required to apply genomic science and associated technologies to improve the understanding of health and disease in diverse populations is undeniable todays. In fact, identify individuals and populations who are at risk for developing specific diseases such as NTDs, and to better understand underlying genetic and environmental contributions to risk could greatly contribute in finding sustainable responses. And the large diversity of African continent that constitute genetic complexity represents an enormous opportunity to utilize such approaches to benefit African populations and to inform global health.

The most involved institution in the training of human resources in genomic are Pan African based in South Africa and Nord Africa. Few are developing in west Africa mainly in Nigeria, Ghana and recently introduced in Mali.

6.1 H3Africa

The Human Heredity and Health in Africa (H3Africa) constitute one of the largest consortium with the objectives to facilitate fundamental research into diseases on the African continent, while also developing infrastructure, resources, training, and ethical guidelines to support a sustainable African research enterprise. By his constitution, H3Africa is led by African scientists, for the African people. Today, H3Africa initiative consists of 48 African projects that include different data set from population-based genomic studies of common, non-communicable disorders such as heart and renal disease to communicable diseases such as tuberculosis. Those studies are designed by African scientists with the objective to identify hereditary and environmental contributions to health and disease. While H3Africa is working mainly in developing African scientist's capacity, the consortium is also committed to support many crucial capacity building elements, such as ethical, legal, and social implications research; training and capacity building for bioinformatics; capacity for biobanking; and coordination and networking.

As a continental consortium, today H3Africa constitutes as one of the most important supporting institutions to African researchers and also contributing to the establishment of effective collaborations among African researchers. Through these different collaborations, the consortium is able to generate specific and large data set in relation to the global health. The consortium is supporting different initiative in Africa such the West African Center of Excellence for Global Health Bioinformatics Research Training in Mali, the Eastern Africa Network for Bioinformatics Training (EANBIT), the Collaborative African Genomics Network" (CAfGEN) and the Integrated approach to the identification of genetic determinants of susceptibility to trypanosomiasis (TrypanoGEN) in Uganda.

H3Africa is also collaborating with the African Center of Excellence for Genomics of Infectious Diseases (ACEGID) at Redeemer's University in partnership with academic, clinical, and research institutions in Nigeria, Sierra-Leone, and Senegal to develop African research capacity in genomics by building a critical mass of well-trained scientists.

In order to boost the genomic concept and interest African scientists to this revolutionary scientific area, a group of stakeholders from the H3BiotNet (Pan African Bioinformatics Network for H3Africa) and the African Society of Human Genetic launched in 2016 in Dakar in Senegal, the African Genomic Medicine Training initiative called AGMT.

The African Genomic Medicine Training Initiative (AGMT) was initiated by a Working Group made up of volunteers from across the globe with a clear vision to "*increased effectiveness of Health Care in Africa through the application of Genomic Medicine*". This initiative includes several mission:

Design and develop Genomic Medicine training for African-based healthcare professionals.
Develop competency-based Genomic Medicine curriculum for healthcare workers in Africa.
Develop and implement flagship training courses based on the collaboratively developed curricula.
The first iteration was run in 2017 with 19 classrooms in 11 countries, 1 online class, and 225 students registered.
The second iteration is running from March to July 2019 as a professional development course.

The purpose of this Professional Development Course is to provide genomics and genetics education to nurses based in Africa emphasizing the practical application of content into learners' current settings and roles. In addition to contributing increasing knowledge in the genetics of African health issues, this second iteration of the AGMT initiative aim to develop skills in Genetic counseling, Community engagement/Ethical conduct in research, and patient care and development of health promotion material. Therefore, this course seeks to support improved Genetics & Genomics knowledge, attitudes and skills for genomic medicine in Africa.

6.2 Genomics Africa

Genomic Africa is a training program organized by the Kwazulu-Natal Research Innovation and Sequencing Platform (KRISP) with the aim of "*Bringing genomic technologies to Africa to fight our great challenges: loss of biodiversity, famine, migration and diseases*."

As a Flagship program of the South African Medical Research Council (SAMRC), KRIS develops collaboration with DIPLOMICS ASSOCIATED LABORATORIES which is a South African Research Infrastructure Roadmap (SARIR) program of the Department of Science and Technology (DST). To reach his mention, different training programs are developed and run each year at KRISP Genomics Africa targeting several diseases including tropical neglected disease as well as the development of new technologies to help in Africa including Microbiome and Metagenomics Sequencing with Illumina and Nanopore.

There are others genomic training initiatives developed and running in Africa, and even not targeting specifically neglected tropical disease are greatly contributing to human resources strengthening. By helping strengthen human capacity in genomic area, they may help answering how African scientists are prepared to tackle the NTDs in the context of genomic era.

6.3 DELGEME

The Developing Excellence in Leadership and Genetics Training for Malaria Elimination in sub-Saharan Africa (DELGEME) is a new training programme sponsored by the Wellcome Trust Developing Excellence in Leadership, Training and Science Africa (DELTAS Africa) initiative in partnership with the Department of International Development (DFID) and the Alliance for

Accelerating Excellence in Science in Africa (AESA). Led by the University of Science Techniques and Technologies of Bamako Mali (USTTB), this genetic and genomic training program is partnering with the Medical Research Council (MRC) Unit in The Gambia, The United States Army Medical Research Directorate (USAMRD-K)/KEMRI Kenya, The Noguchi Memorial Institute for Medical Research (NMIMR)-Navrongo Health Research Centre, Ghana, The National Institute of Medical Research (NIMR) Tanzania, Université des Sciences de la Santé of Libreville, Gabon, Benhard-Nocht Institute for Tropical Medicine (BNITM) Germany/Kumasi Centre for Collaborative Research (KCCR) Ghana, and the University of Oxford/Wellcome Trust Sanger Institute UK. In collaboration with MalariaGEN (www.malariagen.net) and the Plasmodium Diversity Network, The DELGEME program aims to enrich the pool of African Scientists working in African institutions with relevant expertise to leverage big genetics and genomics data in the drive for malaria elimination in sub-Saharan Africa.

In order to reach this objective DELGEME aim to:

To train, retain, and develop Graduates, Doctoral, and Post-doctoral fellows on genomics and bioinformatics across malaria endemic countries.

To develop programs to enhance the understanding and dissemination of genetic data relevant to malaria interventions and eradication program.

Short-term training will be delivered for various trainees including public health officers on genetics, clinical studies, ethics, grant writing, grant management, leadership development, etc.

Formal long-term curricula (big data science, biostatistics, health informatics, genomics, cell biology, molecular biology, and bioinformatics) will be designed and implemented with contribution and oversight from a wide range of local and International Faculty and relevant advisory boards.

DELGEME
Training Leaders for a Malaria-free Africa

6.4 Others genomic training institutions/programs in Africa

Interestingly from last year, genomic education is progressively taking off in Africa. Indeed, many genomic training programs at the countries or regional level are entering in operational phase. Many of them are mainly supported by H3ABioNet which organizes a variety of high quality courses and training events covering various aspects of bioinformatics from general introductory topics to more specialized ones such Next Generation Sequencing and Genome Wide Association Studies analyses. Indeed, H3ABioNet is comprised of 28 Nodes distributed among 17 countries, 16 of which are African.

7. Conclusions

Genomic is a rapidly evolving medical field relying on technological advances and with a direct effect on disease treatment, control, and elimination including such neglected tropical disease. Nevertheless, in Africa, the introduction, the development, and the application of genomic are variously appreciated. Interestingly, there are institutions greatly introduced in genomic era and they are working to spread the knowledge to the rest of the African continent as pioneers with support from some North European and American institutions. Hence, even there is still limit critical mass of African scientists well trained in this new scientific domain to contribute to the diseases control and elimination in general and neglected tropical disease in particular, there is room of hope since there is positive signal within the continent. However, this provided the strongest possible argument in favor of working together in south-south collaboration way on steps to bridge this genomic divide. The challenge exists but still remain surmountable.

Conflict of interest

There is no conflict of interest.

Author details

Issiaka Soulama
National Centre for Training and Malaria Research, Ouagadougou, Burkina Faso

*Address all correspondence to: soulamacnrfp@gmail.com

References

[1] Hotez PJ, Kamath A. Neglected tropical diseases in sub-saharan Africa: Review of their prevalence, distribution, and disease burden. PLoS Neglected Tropical Diseases. 2009;**3**(8):e412

[2] Hotez PJ, Alvarado M, Basáñez MG, Bolliger I, Bourne R, Boussinesq M, et al. The global burden of disease study 2010: Interpretation and implications for the neglected tropical diseases. PLoS Neglected Tropical Diseases. 2014;**8**(7):e2865

[3] Chan M. Ten Years in Public Health, 2007-2017: Report. Geneva: World Health Organization; 2017

[4] Centers for Disease Control and Prevention Neglected Tropical Diseases. 2017. Available from: https://www.cdc.gov/globalhealth/ntd/diseases/index.html [Accessed: 15 June 2017]

[5] Rosenberg M, Utzinger J, Addiss DG. Preventive chemotherapy versus innovative and intensified disease Management in Neglected Tropical Diseases: A distinction whose shelf life has expired. PLoS Neglected Tropical Diseases. 2016;**10**(4):e0004521

[6] Hotez PJ, Molyneux DH, Fenwick A, Kumaresan J, Ehrlich Sachs S, Sachs JD, et al. Control of neglected tropical diseases. New England Journal of Medicine. 2007;**357**:1018-1027

[7] Hotez PJ, Molyneux DH, Fenwick A, Ottesen E, Ehrlich Sachs S, Sachs JD. Incorporating a rapid-impact package for neglected tropical diseases with programs for HIV/AIDS, tuberculosis, and malaria. PLoS Medicine. 2006;**3**:e102

[8] Hotez PJ. The neglected tropical diseases and their devastating health and economic impact on the member nations of the Organization of the Islamic Conference. PLoS Neglected Tropical Diseases. 2009;**3**:e539

[9] Molyneux DH. The 'neglected tropical diseases': Now a brand identity, responsibilities, context and promise. Parasites Vectors. 2012:5-23. DOI: 10.1186/1756-3305-5-23

[10] WHO. Roadmap accelerating work to overcome the global impact of neglected tropical diseases. 2012. 42 p

[11] Mackey TK, Liang BA. Threats from emerging and re-emerging neglected tropical diseases (NTDs). Infection Ecology & Epidemiology. 2012;**2**:75-88. DOI: 10.3402/iee.v2i0.18667

[12] Pappaioanou M, Spencer H. "One health" initiative and ASPH. Public Health Reports. 2008;**123**:261

[13] Lee K, Brumme ZL. Operationalizing the one health approach: The global governance challenges. Health Policy and Planning. 2013;**28**:778-785. DOI: 10.1093/heapol/czs127

[14] Kaplan B, Kahn LH, Monath TP, Woodall J. "ONE HEALTH" and parasitology. Parasites & Vectors. 2009;**2**:36. DOI: 10.1186/1756-3305-2-36

[15] McCarter JP. Genomic filtering: an approach to discovering novel antiparasitics. Trends in Parasitology. 2004;**20**:462-468

[16] Foster JM et al. Mining nematode genome data for novel drug targets. Trends in Parasitology. 2005;**21**:101-104

[17] Mitreva M et al. Comparative genomics of nematodes. Trends in Genetics. 2005;**21**:573-581

Chapter 9

Epidemiology and Ecology of Leishmaniasis

Tonay Inceboz

Abstract

Leishmaniasis is the third most important vector-borne disease after malaria and lymphatic filariasis. It is common disease in all over the world. The vector for leishmaniasis is *Phlebotomus* and there have found around 20 different types of this vector. There are different clinical forms under the name of leishmaniasis such as kala-azar, dum-dum fever, white leprosy, espundia, pian bois, chiclero's ulcer, uta. Environmental factors leading to climate changes and global warming are major risk factors for the spreading of the disease. *Leishmania* spp. to prevent the spread of the definitive host and intermediate hosts is difficult compared to *Plasmodium* spp. Therefore; leishmaniasis disease will retain its importance for many years.

Keywords: leishmaniasis, neglected tropical diseases, vector-borne disease, epidemiology, ecology

1. Introduction

This fact is mainly due to the presence of many different species of *leishmania*, its vectors and hosts in different parts of the world. More than 20 pathologic species of *leishmania* and over 30 species of *Phlebotomus*—the vector- are known worldwide (**Figure 1**, **Table 1**).

On the other hand, deterioration of the eco-systems by human beings also contribute to the spread of the disease in the world.

Leishmaniasis has four clinical forms. These are cutaneous leishmaniasis (CL, local—LCL or diffuse—DCL), mucocutaneous leishmaniasis (MCL), visceral leishmaniasis (VL), post-kala-azar dermal leishmaniasis (PKDL), (**Table 1**).

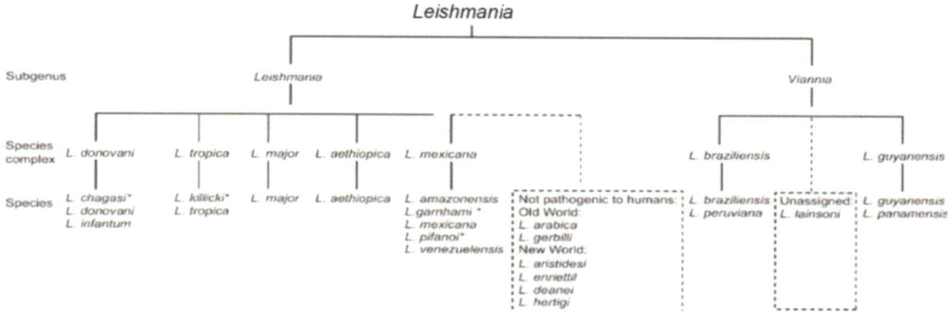

Figure 1.
Taxonomy of leishmania *family [1].*

Subgenus	L. (Leishmania)	L. (Leishmania)	L. (Viannia)	L. (Viannia)
Old World	*L. donovani*	*L. major*		
	L. infantum	*L. tropica*		
		L. killicki[a]		
		L. aethiopica		
		L. infantum		
New World	*L. infantum*	*L. infantum*	*L. braziliensis*	*L. braziliensis*
		L. mexicana	*L. guyanensis*	*L. panamensis*
		L. pifanoi[a]	*L. panamensis*	
		L. venezuelensis	*L. shawi*	
		L. garnhami[a]	*L. naïffi*	
		L. amazonensis	*L. lainsoni*	
			L. lindenbergi	
			L. peruviana	
			L. colombiensis[b]	
Principal tropism	Viscerotropic	Dermotropic	Dermotropic	Mucotropic

[a]*Species status is under discussion.*
[b]*Taxonomic position is under discussion.*

Table 1.
Leishmania *found in humans [1].*

In this section we aimed to reveal the epidemiologic analysis of different types of leishmaniasis in all over the world in every aspect.

2. Geographic distribution and incidence

Leishmaniasis, as being one of the world's most neglected diseases, affects mainly the poor, developing countries; 350 million people are thought to be at risk of contracting leishmaniasis. It is estimated that approximately 12 million men are ill and 2 million new cases occur annually [1, 2].

With new epidemics occurring in endemic areas and the spread of leishmaniasis to previously free areas because of migration, tourism, and military activities. Leishmaniasis is a disease of the poor, occurring mostly in remote rural villages with poor housing and little or no access to modern health-care facilities. In endemic areas, diagnosis of any form of leishmaniasis puts a huge financial strain on an already meagre financial resource at both the individual and community levels [3].

Visceral leishmaniasis: approximately 90% of new cases occur in the world's cases of India, Bangladesh, Nepal, Ethiopia, Sudan and Brazil are seen. The annual number of cases worldwide has been estimated to be visceral leishmaniasis, between 200,000 and 400,000. The two important causative agents of visceral leishmaniasis (VL), namely *Leishmania* (L) *donovani* and *L. infantum*, cause significant health problems [1, 4].

Visceral leishmaniasis (VL), also known as "kala azar," is caused by parasites of the *L. donovani* complex in some parts of the world. The *L. donovani* complex can be found throughout Asia, North Africa, Latin America and Southern Europe, affecting mostly vulnerable and uncared populations. As being the most severe form, VL is almost always fatal if left untreated. It is characterized by undulating fever, loss of weight, splenomegaly, hepatomegaly and/or lymphadenopathies and anemia *L. infantum*, the other causative agent of VL, is found in Southern Europe, North Africa and West and Central Asia [1, 5].

Post-kala-azar dermal leishmaniasis (PKDL) is another clinical composition of kala azar and it is seen in all areas endemic for *L. donovani*. It especially comments in East Africa and on the Indian subcontinent with a prevalence of 50 and 10%, respectively [1, 6].

Cutaneous leishmaniasis: approximately 90% of the world's cases of Afghanistan, Pakistan, Sudan, Syria, Saudi Arabia, Algeria, Iran, Iraq, is seen in Brazil and Peru. The annual number of cases worldwide has been estimated to be visceral leishmaniasis, cutaneous leishmaniasis: between 700,000 and 1.2 million [1]. Old World species: *L. major*, *L. infantum*, and *L. tropica*, New World species, such as, *L. amazonensis*, *L. chagasi*, *L. mexicana*, *L. viannia* (V) *naiffi*, *L.* (V.) *braziliensis*, and *L.* (V.) *guyanensis* [6, 7]. Antroponotic cutaneous leishmaniasis (ACL) is caused by most *Leishmania* species, occur in most subtropical and tropical regions (for example, *L. major* from Africa and Asia, and *L. mexicana* from Central and South America), and by many species in the subgenus *Viannia*, which are limited to Latin America (for example, *L. (V) brasiliensis*) [6].

Old World cutaneous leishmaniasis caused by *L. tropica* (seen particularly in the Mediterranean Basin, the Middle East, Pakistan and India) and *L. infantum*, (found sporadically in the Middle East, South Russia, and rural regions of Africa). New World cutaneous leishmaniasis, caused by *L. brazilensis* and *L. mexicana* is seen in Mexica and South America. Leishmaniasis exists on every continent except Australia, the Pacific Islands and Antarctica. The parasites that cause leishmaniasis are found in 98 countries around the world [7].

L. tropica, *L. major*, *L. aethiopica* and *L. infantum* causes Old World cutaneous leishmaniasis. *Leishmania tropica* is mainly seen in urban areas and causes ACL. Related vectors are *Phlebotomus sergenti* and *Phlebotomus papatasii*. Lesions are generally dry and remain without ulceration. During the course lesions change to papules [1, 8].

L. tropica is found in urban areas. It causes ACL via the vectors *Phlebotomus sergenti* and *Phlebotomus papatasii*. The lesions are dry and stay for a long period of time without ulceration. Thereafter, painless lesions as papules, tubercles or nodules subside without scarring in 9–12 months [8].

L. major infections generally cause wet lesions in habitants of rural areas. Incubation period is less than 4 months. Lesions are usually seen on the legs. They start as acute papillary infection in the bite area and advances into pustular ulcers in 1–3 weeks. The infection is categorized as "zoonotic cutaneous leishmaniasis (ZCL)" due to the transmission to rodents, dogs via *Phlebotomus papatasi* [9].

L. infantum often causes small (0.5–1 cm), solitary ulcers on the face [10].

L. aetropica lesions are seen in the mouth and nose with local or wide spread dermal involvement. Lesions rarely become ulcerated. Healing may take 1–3 years or more [11].

L. braziliensis, *L. mexicana*, *L. amazoensis*, *L. guyanensis*, *L. panamensis* and *L. peruviana* cause New World cutaneous leishmaniasis [8, 12].

The disease caused by *L. braziliensis* is named "espundia." The infection leads to metastatic lesions, damages and deformation of the cartilage and soft tissues by affecting buccal and nasal mucosa [13].

L. mexicana causes usually solitary, painless lesions in the pinna. It leads to chronic lesions in the pinna called "chiclero's ulcer" [14].

L. guyanensis infection is consisted of flat ulcerative plaques with leakage in whole body. The lesion is called "pianbois" in Uruguay and Venezuella [15].

L. amazonensis causes solitary or multiple lesions with rarely spontaneous remission. It is rare in humans [8].

L. peruviana infection causes solitary or multiple painless dermal lesions they usually subsided spontaneously in 4–5 months. This infection is called uta [16].

Lesions of *L. panamensis* are ulcers without spontaneous improvement the reservoirs are dogs and monkeys [12].

L. venezuelensis generally causes solitary painless nodular lesion. [12, 17].

L. garnhami usually causes solitary or multiple lesions and may spontaneously be healed in 6 months [12].

The Eastern Hemisphere (Old World): leishmaniasis is found in some parts of Asia, the Middle East, Africa (especially in the tropical region and North Africa), and Southern Europe.

The Western Hemisphere (New World), leishmaniasis is found in some parts of Mexico, Central America, and South America. It is not found in Chile or Uruguay.

Leishmaniasis is seen in most tropical and subtropical regions with climate, mainly in South and Central America, Africa, Asia, and Southern Europe. The leishmaniasis is considered as one of the neglected tropical diseases (NTD) (**Figures 2** and **3**) [18].

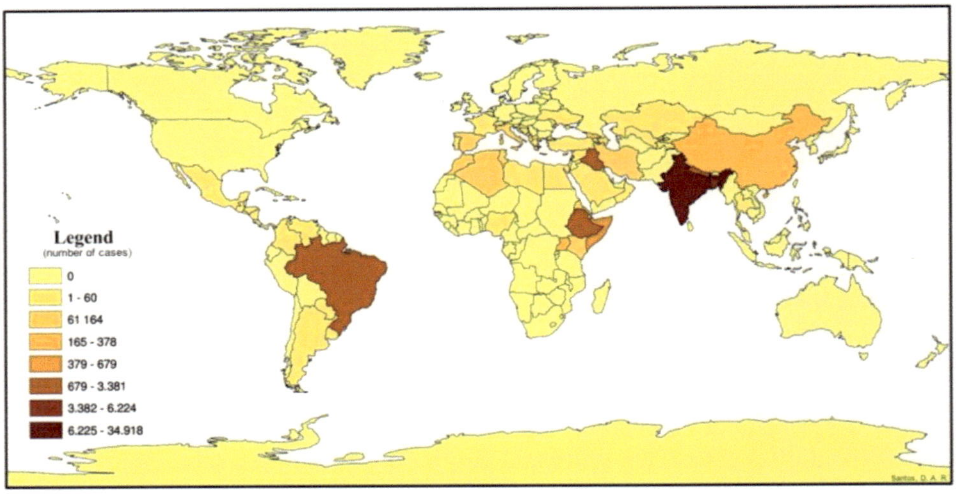

Figure 2.
World VL distribution in the last 10 years [19].

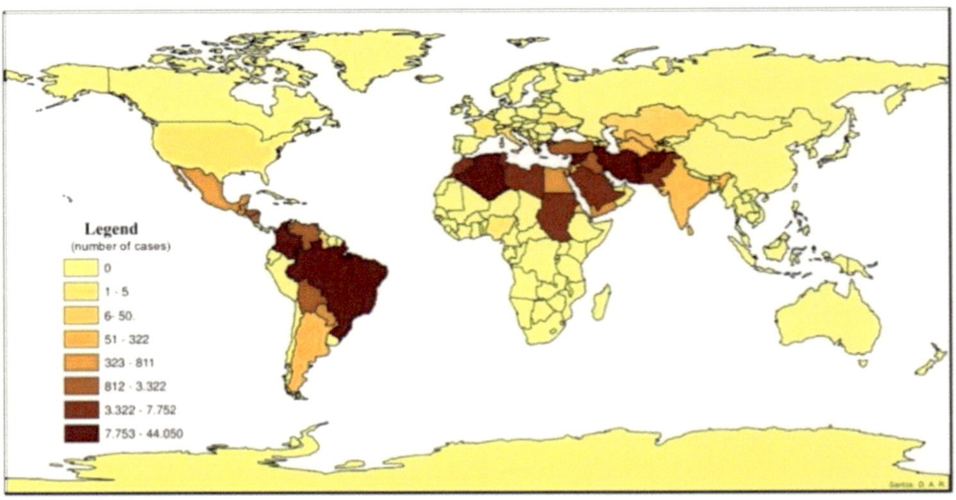

Figure 3.
World CL distribution in the last 10 years [19].

3. Epidemiology of leishmaniasis according to vector

a. *Phlebotomus* spp. (sandfly). (Old World).

b. *Lutzomyia* spp. (New World).

Humidity and moisture, whether from rainfall or in the soil, have often been identified as important for the sandfly, with humidity influencing breeding and resting [6].

Sandflies belonging to either *Phlebotomus* spp. (Old World) or *Lutzomyia* spp. (New World) are the primary vectors; domestic dogs, rodents, sloths, and opossums are amongst a long list of mammals that are either incriminated or suspected reservoir hosts [1, 21, 22]. Most of its foci in the Old World have a Mediterranean climate and sand fly vectors, usually *Phlebotomus* (Larroussius) species, *Phlebotomus* species (*P. papatasi*, *P. sergenti*, *Phlebotomus alexandri*, *P. tobbi*, *Phlebotomus syriacus*, *Phlebotomus neglectus*, *Phlebotomus perfiliewi*, *Phlebotomus galilaeus*, *Phlebotomus transcaucasicus*, and *Phlebotomus halepensis*) two *Sergentomyia* species (*Sergentomyia theodori* and *Sergentomyia dentata*), (*Phlebotomus ariasi* and *Phlebotomus perniciosus*, *Phlebotomus longicuspis*) can diapauses for human visceral leishmaniasis [21–24].

In contrast to malaria, there is little evidence for the effect of vector control in leishmaniasis because terrestrial habitat of *Phlebotomus* is mostly unknown.

4. Host

4.1 Human

Leishmania species are transmitted to human via vectors, blood transfusion, organ transplantation or vertically via transplacental route. Other factors that cause the transmission of the disease are contact with contaminated materials or needle stick injuries in the labs [25–27].

Leishmania-infected humans especially in poor socioeconomic conditions play a pivotal role as a reservoir in transmission of the agent to vectors or to other hosts. In another words, one can say that human beings contribute the disease transmission by themselves [26, 27]. Poor living conditions in adobe, wooden houses, barns create a tendency towards an increase of vectors [27–29].

In all three clinical types of *Leishmania* spp., antimonials (sodium stibogluconate [SSG]), miltefosin (MIL), amfoterisin B (AmB) veparomomisin (PMM)) are being used [30]. Children and people with immune suppression, HIV infection or malignant diseases cause rapid spread of leishmaniasis. Apart from these, undiagnosed or untreated infected people create an important risk factor. Especially drug resistance and high expense of the medication cause insufficient treatment [27–29]. The first drug resistance was reported in VL treatment against SSG and against MIL, in India and Nepal, respectively [31–33]. Later, resistance against MIL was also reported in one patient with HIV and another two patients with Indian origin [34, 35].

Verma et al. showed that the effectiveness of PMM was decreased by 6 times for the promastigote forms of *L. donavani* [36]. Invasion of macrophages by PMM-R parasites led to increased nitric oxide (NO), whereas the levels of reactive oxygen species (ROS) remained unchanged. This finding shows resistance of *Leishmania* spp. against PMM [36]. Similarly, Deep et al., reported high recurrence rates in patients with VL and PKDL when treated with MIL [37].

In conclusion, due to immune problems of the patient, co-existence of other diseases, inappropriate use of the drugs during the medical treatment of leishmaniasis, "drug resistance" may occur via gene over-expression, deletion, single nucleotide

*Leishmania*species	Disease	Countries (suspected)	Landscapes	Reservoir hosts	Vector
Old World					
L. donovani	AVL, DCL, CL	Northeast India, Nepal, Bangladesh, (Bhutan), Sri Lanka, Republic of China, Sudan, Ethiopia, (Chad), (Yemen), Kenya	Rural, peri-domestic	Human anthroponosis	*P. (Eu.) argentipes, P. (La.) orientalis, P. (Sy.) martini*
L. donovani	AVL	People's Republic of China	Rural, peri-domestic	Unknown	*P. (Pa.) alexandri, P. (Ad.)* species
L. donovanib (L. archibaldi)	AVL, ZVL, ML	Sudan, Ethiopia, (Chad), (Yemen)	Rural, *Acacia—Balanites* forest	Human anthroponosis	*P. (Larroussius) orientalis*
L. donovanib (L. archibaldi)	AVL, DCL	Sudan, Ethiopia, Kenya, (Uganda)	Rural, savannatermite mounds	Human anthroponosis	*P. (Sy.) martini*
L. infantum	ZVL, ZCL	Med Europe, North Africa, Southwest Asia, People's Republic of China	Rural, peri-domestic	Domestic dog, wild canids, domestic cat	*P. (La.) ariasi, perniciosus*
L. infantumc (L. chagasi)	VL, CL	Latin America: not Peru or Guianas	Rural, peri-domestic	Domestic dog, wild canids	*Lu. (L.) longipalpis*
L. major	ZCL	North Africa, Ethiopia, Kenya, Sudan, Meadle Asia India	Peri-domestic	Human anthroponosis	*P. papatasi, P. duboscqi*
Le. (Le.) tropica	ACL	North Africa, Middle East, Iran, Afghanistan	Urban	Peridomestic, including suburbs; human	*P. (Paraphlebotomus) sergenti*
Le. (Le.) tropicac (Le. (Le.) killicki)	ZCL	North Africa, MiddleEast, Sub-Saharan Africa	Rural	Rockyarid; hyraxes, Rodents	*P. (Adlerius) arabicus P. (La.) guggisbergi*
Le. (Le.) aethiopica;	ZCL,DCL, ML	Ethiopia, Kenya	Rural, Rocky highlands	Hyraxes	*P. (La.) longipes P. (La.) pedifer*
New World					
Leishmania (Leishmania) infantum	ZVL, ZCL	Latin America: not Peru, Guianas	Peridomestic, including suburbs	Domestic dog	*Lutzomyia (Lutzomyia) longipalpis*s.l.
Leishmania (Viannia) braziliensis	ZCL, ML	East of Andes: not Guyana, Suriname	Peridomestic, silvatic	Rodents, marsupials, dog	*L. (Psychodopygus) wellcomei L. (Nyssomyia) neivai L. (Ny.) whitmani*

*Leishmania*species	Disease	Countries (suspected)	Landscapes	Reservoir hosts	Vector
Le. (*V.*) *braziliensis*	ZCL, ML	West of Andes, northern Venezuela: not El Salvador	Peridomestic, silvatic	Rodents, marsupials, dog	*L.* (*Pifanomyia*) *ovallesi*
Le. (*V.*) *peruviana*	ZCL, ML	Peru	Peridomestic, silvatic	Rodents, marsupials, dog	*L.* (*He.*) *peruensis*s.l. *L.* (*Pf.*) *verrucarum*s.l.
Le. (*V.*) *guyanensis*	ZCL, ML	East of Andes: not Paraguay	Silvatic	Arboreal edentates, others	*L.* (*Ny.*) *umbratilis*
Le. (*V.*) *panamensis*	ZCL, ML	West of Andes, northern Venezuela: not Mexico, Belize, El Salvador	Silvatic	Arboreal edentates, others	*L.* (*Ny.*) *trapidoi L.* (*Ny.*) *ylephiletor L.* (*Ny.*) *edentula L.* (*Tricholateralis*) *gomezi*
Le. (*V.*) *shawi*	ZCL	Brazil	Silvatic	Arboreal	*L.* (*Trichophoromyia*) *ubiquitalis L.* (*Pf.*) *nuneztovari*
Le. (*V.*) *lainsoni*	ZCL	Bolivia, Peru, Brazil, French Guiana, Suriname	Silvatic	Rodent *Agouti paca*	*L.* (*Trichophoromyia*) *ubiquitalis L.* (*Pf.*) *nuneztovari*
Le. (*V.*) *colombiensis*	ZCL	Panama, Colombia, Venezuela	Silvatic	*Choloepushoffmanni*	*L.* (*He.*) *hartmanni*
Le. (*V.*) *naiffi*	ZCL	Brazil, French Guiana, Panama	Silvatic	*Dasypusnovemcinctus*	*L.* (*Ps.*) *ayrozai* and other species *L.* (*Ny.*) *trapidoic*
Le. (*Le.*) *amazonensis*	ZCL, DCL	East of Andes: not Guyana, Paraguay	Silvatic, non-climax forest	Terrestrial rodents, Marsupials	*L.* (*Ny.*) *flaviscutellata*
Le. (*Le.*) *mexicana*	ZCL, DCL, ML	West of Andes, southern United States: not Peru	Silvatic, non-climax forest	Terrestrial rodents, Marsupials	*L.* (*Ny.*) *olmecaolmeca*
Le. (*Le.*) *venezuelensis*	ZCL, DCL	Northern Venezuela	Silvatic	Unknown	*L.* (*Ny.*) *olmecabicolor*

Abbreviations: TC, transmission cycle; A, anthroponotic; Z, zoonotic; V, visceral; C, cutaneous; M, mucosal; D, diffuse; L, leishmaniasis. P., Phlebotomus; Pa., Paraphlebotomus; Pf., Pifanomyia; Sy., Synphlebotomus La., Larroussius; Lu., Lutzomyia.

Table 2.
Disease types and transmission cycles of leishmaniasis worldwide [6, 20, 21].

polymorphisms generating stop codons or amplification of sets of genes [38–40]. This very important for epidemiological standpoint and thus proper use of drugs when needed should be stressed, and also new drug formulations and/or vaccine should be investigated.

Technological advances let the people travel all over the world. This may cause vectored spread or spread directly by infected people [41].

4.2 Dogs

Dogs are very important in terms of the epidemiology of leishmaniasis. All forms of leishmaniasis namely cutaneous, mucocutaneous and visceral types may be found in dogs. Since the infected dogs are important reservoir of the disease, their controls and treatments are mandatory for the disease control. Dogs as pets are being controlled by vets however stray or wild dogs, fox species like *Lycalopex vetulus* [42], *Cerdocyonthous* [43] may cause outbreaks. Dogs are natural hosts for *L. infantum*, *L. chagasi*, *L. tropica* and *L. peruviana* as well as being infected by them. Especially they are endemic in dogs in Mediterranean region, Asia and Latin America. *Leishmania infantum* is the causative agent of visceral leishmaniasis and it is prevalent especially in Mediterranean region. Vectors for this type are *Phlebotomus ariasi*, *P. major*, *P. perniciosus*, *P. longicuspis*, *P. chiensis*, *P. mongolensis*, *P. papatasi* [44, 45]. In the same region, the causative agent of zoonotic cutaneous leishmaniasis is *L. tropica* and the vectors are *P. perfilievi*, *P. papatasi* and *P. sergenti* [1, 46]. In South America, the causative agent of canine cutaneous leishmaniasis is *L. chagasi* and the vectors are *Lu. longipalpalis*, *Lu. evansi*, *Lu. gomezi* [1].

4.3 Rodents

Comparing to dogs, eradication of the infectious agent of leishmaniasis from the rodents is more difficult and even sometimes impossible.

Different rodents such as *Didelphis albiventris* (opossum), *Mus musculus* (domestic mouse), *Microtus socialis*, *Rattusrattus* (black rat), *Cercomys cunicularius* (wild rat), *Mesocricetus auratus* (Syrian hamsters) in America, Africa and Asia lead to spread of leishmaniasis [47–51].

Phlebotomus papatasi, vector of *L. tropica*, transmitted cutaneous leishmaniasis to small rodents such as *Psammomys obesus* (Israel), *Meriones crassus* (Israel), *Meriones libycus* (Iran), *Rhombomys opimus* (Iran), *Rhombomys opimus* (Iran), *Meriones sacramenti* (Egypt) [9].

Rattus rattus and *Rattus norvegicus* have been found naturally infected with *L. infantum* in the Mediterranean and in Next Orient endemic areas (**Table 2**) [49, 52, 53].

5. Transmission cycle

There are two different types of transmission;

1. In many geographic areas, infected people are not needed to sustain the transmission cycle of the parasite in nature; transmission cycle continue via the infected animals (rodents or dogs, felines). *Leishmania* infection in reservoir animals are specifically named; if it is in dogs, it is named as canine leishmaniasis whereas in cats, it is called feline leishmaniasis dogs species of *Leishmania* species in the reservoir in animals, canine leishmaniasis, which is in feline called leishmaniasis. *L. infantum* is the most common and important cause of canine leishmaniasis worldwide. The **zoonotic transmission** of *L.*

infantum, from canine to humans, is not only in the Mediterranean region where it may have originated, but also it may be found in many of the drier regions of Latin America. *Leishmania* species reported from dogs include *L. mexicana*, *L. donovani*, and *L. braziliensis*. These *Leishmania* species are occasionally reported from the cats. Cats are at risk of infection especially in areas where these parasites are endemic [6, 54, 55].

2. In some parts of the world, infected people are needed to sustain the cycle; this kind of transmission (human—*Phlebotomus*—human) is called **anthroponotic transmission**.

Full knowledge on these two transmission cycles is very important in effective prevention of leishmaniasis [54, 55].

6. Effect of deteriorated eco-system on spread of leishmaniasis

Unlike other parasites, it is extremely difficult to eradicate whole kinds of species of *Leishmania* in nature. This is contrary to some other parasites. As example *Plasmodium vivax* is specific to human, thus it can be eradicated by vector control. However, this is not the case for *Leishmania* spp. [54, 55].

There are many check points to establish the control of the disease. Firstly, all patients with leishmaniasis should be properly treated. *Leishmania* transmission is dependent on the togetherness of contaminated sandflies with the reservoir hosts, and humans. Additionally, climatic and environment factors are important, too.

As the development of chemical insecticides use such as dichlorodiphenyltrichloroethane (DDT) against mosquito was a key component of the eradication, similarly they were proposed to have an effect on the sandflies, vectors of visceral leishmaniasis [56–58]. Since DDT use is found to be harmful to the environment and people, its use is prohibited by the World Health Organization [59]. At the moment there isn't any strategy to control *Phlebotomine* by using insecticides by governments [60, 61]. Preliminary experiments for developing a vaccine against *Leishmania* spp. was reported [62]. However, the vaccine did not appear to protect against visceral leishmaniasis [63]. fucose-mannose ligand from an extract of *L. donovani* has been used in conjunction with a saponin adjuvant in attempts to vaccine [64]. Further studies are needed to develop an effective vaccine against leishmaniasis.

7. Summary

Leishmaniasis is still an important parasite disease in all over the world. The reasons are presence of many different species of *Leishmania*, and their ability to survive in many different organisms, such as vectors, dogs, rodents, humans. *Leishmania* spp. may cause different clinical scenarios by affecting different tissues and organs. As eukaryotic cells, *Leishmania* spp. can survive in the immune system of the most advanced organism, human. Presence of amastigote forms even in the hosts' defensive cells shows the strength of the parasite.

Leishmaniasis is an important public health problem. Thus, relevant public health policies such as education of the people especially in endemic areas, multidisciplinary approach, diagnosis, treatment will be helpful in the elimination of the disease. Additionally, further epidemiological studies as well as vaccination studies will continue to strive for eradication.

Author details

Tonay Inceboz
Department of Parasitology, Medical Faculty, Dokuz Eylul University, Izmir, Turkey

*Address all correspondence to: tonay.inceboz@gmail.com

References

[1] WHO Expert Committee. Control of the leishmaniasis: Report of a meeting of the WHO Expert Committee on the Control of Leishmaniases, Geneva, 2010; 22-26 March. WHO Technical Report Series; 949:1-186. Available from: http://apps.who.int/iris/bitstream/10665/44412/1/WHO_TRS_949_eng.pdf

[2] Ghaffar A. Microbiology and Immunology Online, Parasıtology—Chapter Two Blood and Tıssue Protozoa Part 1 Trypanosomiasıs and Leishmaniasis. 2013. Available from: http://www.microbiologybook.org/parasitology/blood-proto.htm

[3] Okwor I, Uzonna J. Social and economic burden of human leishmaniasis. The American Journal of Tropical Medicine and Hygiene. 2016;**94**(3):489-493. DOI: 10.4269/ajtmh.15-0408

[4] Zijlstra EE. Visceral leishmaniasis: A forgotten epidemic. Archives of Disease in Childhood. 2016;**101**(6):561-567

[5] Gouzelou E, Haralambous C, Antoniou M, Christodoulou V, Martinković F, Živičnjak T, et al. Genetic diversity and structure in *Leishmania infantum* populations from southeastern Europe revealed by microsatellite analysis. Parasites & Vectors. 2013;**6**:342. DOI: 10.1186/1756-3305-6-342

[6] Ready PD. Biology of phlebotomine sand flies as vectors of disease agents. Annual Review of Entomology. 2013;**58**:227-250. DOI: 10.1146/annurev-ento-120811-153557

[7] de Vries HJ, Reedijk SH, Schallig HD. Cutaneous leishmaniasis: Recent developments in diagnosis and management. American Journal of Clinical Dermatology. 2015;**16**:99-109. DOI: 10.1007/s40257-015-0114-z

[8] Krotoski MJ. Medical Parasitology. 8th ed. London: W.B. Saunders Company; 1999. pp. 147-154

[9] Klaus SN, Frankenburg H, Ingber A. Epidemiology of cutaneous leishmaniosis. Clinical Dermatology. 1999;**17**:257-260. DOI: 10.1016/S0738-081X(99)00043-7

[10] Bensaid M, Guerbouj S, Saghrouni F, Fathallah-Mili A, Guizani I. Occurrence of *Leishmania infantum* cutaneous leishmaniasis in Central Tunisia. Transactions of the Royal Society of Tropical Medicine and Hygiene. 2006;**100**:521-526. DOI: 10.1016/j.trstmh.2005.08.012

[11] Özbel Y, Töz ÖS. Leishmaniosis. In: Özcel MA, editor. Tıbbi Parazit Hastalıkları. 1.Baskı ed. İzmir: Meta Basım Matbacılık Hizmetleri; 2007. pp. 198-230

[12] Achtman JC, Ellis DL, Saylors B, Boh EE. Cutaneous leishmaniasis caused by *Leishmania* (Viannia) panamensis in 2 travelers. JAAD Case Reports. 2016;**2**:95-97. DOI: 10.1016/j.jdcr.2015.11.018

[13] Marsden PD. Mucosal leishmaniasis ("espundia" Escomel, 1911). Transactions of the Royal Society of Tropical Medicine and Hygiene. 1986;**80**:859-876. DOI: 10.1016/0035-9203(86)90243-9

[14] Calvopiña M, Martinez L, Hashiguchi Y. Cutaneous leishmaniasis "chiclero's ulcer" in subtropical Ecuador. The American Journal of Tropical Medicine and Hygiene. 2013;**89**:195-196. DOI: 10.4269/ajtmh.12-0690

[15] Lainson R, Shaw JJ, Ready PD, Miles MA, Póvoa M. Leishmaniasis in Brazil: XVI. Isolation and identification of *Leishmania* species from sandflies, wild mammals and man in north Para

state, with particular reference to *L. braziliensis guyanensis* causative agent of "pian-bois". Transactions of the Royal Society of Tropical Medicine and Hygiene. 1981;**75**:530-536. DOI: 10.1016/0035-9203(81)90192-9

[16] Llanos-Cuentas EA, Roncal N, Villaseca P, Paz L, Ogusuku E, Pérez JE, et al. Natural infections of *Leishmania* peruviana in animals in the Peruvian Andes. Transactions of the Royal Society of Tropical Medicine and Hygiene. 1999;**93**:15-20. DOI: 10.1016/S0035-9203(99)90163-3

[17] Ovallos FG, Silva YR, Fernandez N, Gutierrez R, Galati EA, Sandoval CM. The sandfly fauna, anthropophily and the seasonal activities of Pintomyia spinicrassa (*Diptera*: *Psychodidae*: *Phlebotominae*) in a focus of cutaneous leishmaniasis in northeastern Colombia. Memórias do Instituto Oswaldo Cruz. 2013;**108**:297-302. DOI: 10.1590/S0074-02762013000300007

[18] WHO. Neglected Tropical Diseases, Hidden Successes, Emerging Opportunities. Geneva: World Health Organization; 2009. p. 59

[19] Aversi-Ferreira RAGMF, Galvão JD, da Silva SF, Cavalcante GF, da Silva EV, Bhatia-Dey N, et al. Geographical and environmental variables of leishmaniasis transmission. In: Claborn DM, editor. Leishmaniasis—Trends in Epidemiology, Diagnosis and Treatment. InTech; 2014. DOI: 10.5772/57546

[20] Pigott DM, Bhatt S, Golding N, Duda KA, Battle KE, Brady OJ, et al. Global distribution maps of the leishmaniases. eLife. 2014;**3**. DOI: 10.7554/eLife.02851

[21] Ready PD. Epidemiology of visceral leishmaniasis. Clinical Epidemiology. 2014;**6**:147-154. DOI: 10.2147/CLEP.S44267

[22] Amro A, Hamdi S, Lemrani M, Idrissi M, Hida M, Rhajaoui M, et al. Moroccan *Leishmania infantum*: Genetic diversity and population structure as revealed by multi-locus microsatellite typing. PLoS ONE. 2013;**8**:e77778. DOI: 10.1371/journal.pone.0077778

[23] Kavur H, Eroglu F, Evyapan G, Demirkazik M, Alptekin D, Koltas IS. Entomological survey for sand fly fauna in imamoglu province (cutaneous leishmaniasis endemic region) of Adana, Turkey. Journal of Medical Entomology. 2015;**52**:813-818. DOI: 10.1093/jme/tjv064

[24] Kasap OE, Belen A, Kaynas S, Simsek FM, Biler L, Ata N, et al. Activity patterns of sand fly (*Diptera*: *Psychodidae*) species and comparative performance of different traps in an endemic cutaneous leishmaniasis focus in cukurova plain, Southern Anatolia, Turkey. Acta Veterinaria. 2008;**78**: 327-335. DOI: 10.2754/avb200978020327

[25] Silva Jde A, Araújo Ide M, Pavanetti LC, Okamoto LS, Dias M. Visceral leishmaniasis and pregnancy in renal transplanted patient: Case report. Jornal Brasileiro de Nefrologia. 2015;**37**:268-270. DOI: 10.5935/0101-2800.20150041

[26] de Silva AA, Silva Filho ÁPE, Sesso Rde C, Esmeraldo Rde M, de Oliveira CM, Fernandes PF, et al. Epidemiologic, clinical, diagnostic and therapeutic aspects of visceral leishmaniasis in renal transplant recipients: Experience from thirty cases. BMC Infectious Diseases. 2015;**25**(15):96. DOI: 10.1186/s12879-015-0852-9

[27] Fishman JA. Infections in immunocompromised hosts and organ transplant recipients: Essentials. Liver Transplantation. 2011;**17**(Suppl 3): S34-S37. DOI: 10.1002/lt.22378

[28] Alvar J, Aparicio P, Aseffa A, Den Boer M, Canavate C, et al. The relationship between leishmaniasis and

AIDS: The second 10 years. Clinical Microbiology Reviews. 2008;**21**:334-359. DOI: 10.1128/CMR.00061-07

[29] van Griensven J, Ritmeijer K, Lynen L, Diro E. Visceral leishmaniasis as an AIDS defining condition: Towards consistency across WHO guidelines. PLoS Neglected Tropical Diseases. 2014;**17**(8):e2916. DOI: 10.1371/journal.pntd.0002916

[30] Croft SL, Coombs GH. Leishmaniasis—Current chemotherapy and recent advances in the search for novel drugs. Trends in Parasitology. 2003;**19**:502-508

[31] Mittal MK, Rai S, Ashutosh, Ravinder, Gupta S, Sundar S, et al. Characterization of natural antimony resistance in *Leishmania donovani* isolates. The American Journal of Tropical Medicine and Hygiene. 2007;**76**(4):681-688

[32] Rijal S, Ostyn B, Uranw S, Rai K, Bhattarai NR, Dorlo TP, et al. Increasing failure of miltefosine in the treatment of Kala-azar in Nepal and the potential role of parasite drug resistance, reinfection, or noncompliance. Clinical Infectious Diseases. 2013;**56**(11):1530-1538. DOI: 10.1093/cid/cit102

[33] Mondelaers A, Sanchez-Cañete MP, Hendrickx S, Eberhardt E, Garcia-Hernandez R, Lachaud L, et al. Genomic and molecular characterization of miltefosine resistance in *Leishmania infantum* strains with either natural or acquired resistance through experimental selection of intracellular amastigotes. PLoS ONE. 2016;**11**(4):e0154101. DOI: 10.1371/journal.pone.0154101

[34] Srivastava S, Mishra J, Gupta AK, Singh A, Shankar P, Singh S. Laboratory confirmed miltefosine resistant cases of visceral leishmaniasis from India. Parasites & Vectors. 2017;**10**(1):49. DOI: 10.1186/s13071-017-1969-z

[35] Cojean S, Houze ÂS, Haouchine D, Huteau F, Lariven S, Hubert V, et al. *Leishmania* resistance to miltefosine associated with genetic marker. Emerging Infectious Diseases. 2012;**18**(4):704-706. DOI: 10.3201/eid1804.110841

[36] Verma A, Bhandari V, Deep DK, Sundar S, Dujardin JC, Singh R, et al. Transcriptome profiling identifies genes/pathways associated with experimental resistance to paromomycin in *Leishmania donovani*. International Journal for Parasitology: Drugs and Drug Resistance. 2017;**7**(3):370-377. DOI: 10.1016/j.ijpddr.2017.10.004

[37] Deep DK, Singh R, Bhandari V, Verma A, Sharma V, Wajid S, et al. Increased miltefosine tolerance in clinical isolates of *Leishmania donovani* is associated with reduced drug accumulation, increased infectivity and resistance to oxidative stress. PLoS Neglected Tropical Diseases. 2017;**11**(6):e0005641. DOI: 10.1371/journal.pntd.0005641

[38] Ponte-Sucre A, Gamarro F, Dujardin J-C, Barrett MP, LoÂpez-VeÂlez R, Garcõ Âa-HernaÂndez R, et al. Drug resistance and treatment failure in leishmaniasis: A 21st century challenge. PLoS Neglected Tropical Diseases. 2017;**11**(12):e0006052. DOI: 10.1371/journal.pntd.0006052

[39] Hefnawy A, Berg M, Dujardin JC, De Muylder G. Exploiting knowledge on *Leishmania* drug resistance to support the quest for new drugs. Trends in Parasitology. 2017;**33**(3):162-174. DOI: 10.1016/j.pt.2016.11.003

[40] Rastrojo A, García-Hernández R, Vargas P, Camacho E, Corvo L, Imamura H, et al. Genomic and transcriptomic alterations in *Leishmania donovani* lines experimentally resistant to antileishmanial drugs. International Journal for Parasitology: Drugs and

Drug Resistance. 2018;**8**(2):246-264. DOI: 10.1016/j.ijpddr.2018.04.002

[41] Kotton CN. Travel and transplantation: Travel-related diseases in transplant recipients. Current Opinion in Organ Transplantation. 2012;**17**:594-600. DOI: 10.1097/MOT.0b013e328359266b

[42] Lund PV. Fortsatte Bemaerkninger over Brasiliensuddö de Dyrskagning. Kongelige Danske Videnskabernes Selskabs Naturvidenskabeligeog Mathematiske Afhandlinger. 1842;**9**:1-136

[43] Lainson R, Elizabeth FR. *Lutzomyia* longipalpis and the eco-epidemiology of American visceral leishmaniasis, with particular reference to Brazil: A review. Memórias do Instituto Oswaldo Cruz. 2005;**100**:811-827. DOI: 10.1590/S0074-02762005000800001

[44] Capelli G. Asymptomatic and symptomatic dogs in endemic areas, their role in the epidemiology of canine leishmaniosis. In: The 2nd Canine Vector-Borne Disease (CVBD) Symposium; Mazara del Vallo, Sicily, Italy; 2007. pp. 58-63. Available from: http://www.cvbd.org/static/documents/digest/CVBD_Easy-to-digest_no_1_leishmaniosis.pdf [Accessed: 14 june 2016]

[45] Baneth G, Koutinas AF, Solano-Gallego L, Bourdeau P, Ferrer L. Canine leishmaniosis—New concepts and insights on an expanding zoonosis: Part one. Trends in Parasitology. 2008;**24**:324-330. DOI: 10.1016/j.pt.2008.04.001

[46] Banuls AL, Hide M, Prugnolle F. *Leishmania* and the leishmaniases: A parasite genetic update and advances in taxonomy, epidemiology and pathogenicity in humans. Advances in Parasitology. 2007;**64**:1-109-455-458. DOI: 10.1016/S0065-308X(06)64001-3

[47] Sherlock IA. Ecological interactions of visceral leishmaniasis in the state of Bahia, Brazil. Memórias do Instituto Oswaldo Cruz. 1996;**91**:671-683. DOI: 10.1590/S0074-02761996000600003

[48] Lainson R. The American leishmaniases: Some observations on their ecology and epidemiology. Transactions of the Royal Society of Tropical Medicine and Hygiene. 1983;**77**:569-596. DOI: 10.1016/0035-9203(83)90185-2

[49] El-Adhami B. Isolation of *Leishmania* from a black rat in the Baghdad area, Iraq. The American Journal of Tropical Medicine and Hygiene. 1976;**25**:759-761

[50] Inceboz T, Lambrecht FY, Eren MŞ, Girginkardeşler N, Bekiş R, Yilmaz O, et al. Evaluation of ^{131}I-pentamidine for scintigraphy of experimentally *Leishmania tropica*-infected hamsters. Journal of Drug Targeting. 2014;**22**:416-420. DOI: 10.3109/1061186X.2013.878943

[51] Pourmohammadi B, Motazedian MH, Kalantari M. Rodent infection with *Leishmania* in a new focus of human cutaneous leishmaniasis, in northern Iran. Annals of Tropical Medicine and Parasitology. 2008;**102**:127-133. DOI: 10.1179/136485908X252223

[52] Pozzio E, Gradoni L, Bettini S, Gramiccia M. Leishmaniasis in Tuscani (Italy) V. Further isolation of *leishmania* from Rattusrattusin the province of Grosseto. Annals of Tropical Medicine and Parasitology. 1981;**75**:393-395 doi.org/10.5169/seals-312840

[53] Papadogiannakis E, Spanakos G, Kontos V, Menounos PG, Tegos N, Vakalis N. Molecular detection of *Leishmania infantum* in wild rodents (*Rattus norvegicus*) in Greece. Zoonoses and Public Health. 2010;**57**:e23-e25. DOI: 10.1111/j.1863-2378.2009.01264.x

[54] Ashford RW. The leishmaniases as model zoonoses. Annals of Tropical Medicine and Parasitology. 1997;**91**: 693-701. DOI: 10.1080/00034989760428

[55] Lukes J, Mauricio IL, Schönian G, Dujardin JC, Soteriadou K, Dedet JP, et al. Evolutionary and geographical history of the *Leishmania donovani* complex with are vision of current taxonomy. Proceedings of the National Academy of Sciences of the United States of America. 2007;**104**:9375-9380. DOI: 10.1073/pnas.0703678104

[56] Deane LM. Leishmaniose visceral no Brasil. Serviço Nacional de Educação Sanitária. 1956:1-162. Available from: http://www.scielo.br/scielo.php?script=sci_nlinks&ref=000065&pid=S0102-311X200800120002400008&lng=en

[57] Deane LM. Epidemiologia e profilaxia do calazaramericano. Revista Brasileira de Malariologia. 1958;**10**:431-450. Available from: http://www.scielo.br/scielo.php?script=sci_nlinks&ref=000022&pid=S0102-311X200800070002600001&lng=en

[58] Alencar JE. Profilaxia do calazar no Ceará Brasil. Revista do Instituto de Medicina Tropical de São Paulo. 1961;**3**:175-180. Available from: http://www.scielosp.org/scieloOrg/php/reflinks.php?refpid=S0034-89101990000500003000003&lng=pt&pid=S0034-89101990000500003

[59] World Health Organization (WHO). Control of Leishmaniasis. Tech Rep Series. 793, Geneva; 1990. 158 pp

[60] Alencar JE. Kala-azar in Brazil. Scientific Reports of the Istituto Superiore di Sanità. 1962;**2**:116-123

[61] Apostila UFPE. Available from: http://www.ufpe.br/biolmol/Leishmanioses-Apostila_on_line/infogerais.htm. 2013;**16**:99-109

[62] Mayrink W, Genero O, Silva JCF, Costa RT, Tafuri WL, Toledo VPCP, et al. Phase I and II open clinical trials of a vaccine against *Leishmania* chagasi infection in dogs. Memórias do Instituto Oswaldo Cruz. 1996;**91**:695-697. DOI: 10.1590/S0074-02761996000600006

[63] Genaro O, Pinto JA, Costa CA, França-Silva JC, Costa RT, Silva JC, et al. Phase III randomized double blind clinical trial on the efficacy of a vaccine against canine visceral leishmaniasis in urban area of Montes Claros, MG, Brazil. Memórias do Instituto Oswaldo Cruz. 1996;**91**(Suppl):166. Available from: http://memorias.ioc.fiocruz.br/component/k2/item/5932-immunology-212-phase-iii-randomized-double-blind-clinical-trial-on-the-efficacy-of-a-vaccine-against-canine-visceral-leishmaniasis-in-urban-area-of-montes-claros-mg-brazil

[64] Silva VO, Borja-Cabrera GP, Correia Pontes NN, Souza EP, Luz KG, Palatinik M, et al. A Phase III trial of efficacy of the FML-vaccine against canine calazar in an endemic area of Brasil (São Gonçalo do Amarante, RN). Vaccine. 2000;**19**:1082-1092. DOI: 10.1016/S0264-410X(00)00339-X